THE
COMPLETE BOOK
OF GINSENG

CONDITIONS OF SALE

IMPORTANT NOTICE

THE
COMPLETE BOOK
OF GINSENG

RICHARD HEFFERN

CELESTIAL ARTS
Millbrae, California

Copyright © 1976 by Richard Heffern

CELESTIAL ARTS
231 Adrian Road
Millbrae, California 94030

First Printing, September 1976
Made in the United States of America

Library of Congress Cataloging in Publication Data

Heffern, Richard
    The complete book of ginseng.

    Bibliography: p.
    Includes index.
    1. Ginseng. 2. Ginseng (in religion, folklore,
etc.) I. Title.
SB295.G5H4   615'.323'687   75-28757
ISBN   0-89087-151-5

1 2 3 4 5 6 7 8 - 83 82 81 80 79 78 77 76

CONTENTS

Introduction

Few plants have enjoyed the amount of esteem, lore, and mystery that is associated with the ginseng plant. In those cultures in which it is used, ginseng holds a prominent and important place as a botanical medicine. In some instances, people have killed to obtain ginseng. A fortune has been paid willingly more than once to obtain a near-perfect root. It is, in general, the most expensive botanical medicine known.

Perhaps, however, it should be emphasized that there are two distinct varieties of ginseng—the ginseng of Asia, *Panax schinseng*, and the North American variety, *Panax quinquefolium*. Numerous minor variations exist in the two species.

This book will attempt to cover the entire subject of ginseng, including the botanical variations, the history and legends surrounding the plant, the many grades of ginseng, methods of cultivation, and recent research findings.

Throughout the book, a careful comparison has been made of Oriental ginseng and North American ginseng for the purpose of finding similarities and differences. One of the most striking results of this comparison is that the native legends concerning Asiatic ginseng resemble the legends of the North American Indians concerning North American ginseng to an extraordinary degree. Assuming that the peoples of Asia and North America had little contact until recent times, it would appear that very similar legends grew up in two areas isolated from each other. For instance, both continents used ginseng as an amulet, alluding to it as a "man-image." Both continents used it as an aphrodisiac and general strengthener, and so on.

One possible explanation for similarities that exist among different cultures in relation to ginseng is that many of these beliefs and uses originated centuries ago among the Turanian shamans that once inhabited Siberia. It has been suggested that the influence of the ancient Turanians gradually diffused across the Bering Strait into North America, and simultaneously into other parts of Asia—into India, Tibet, Nepal, and Mongolia.

This would not only explain similarities in regard to ginseng, but also traditions and practices relating to magic and sorcery. For instance, trance states for the purpose of finding lost articles; the various snake cults in which live snakes are used in ceremonies and rituals; and similarities of amulets and talismans can be found among many isolated cultures throughout the world. For example, amulets made in the fourth and fifth centuries in Greece bear close resemblance to amulets made in Arabia and China at that time.

Although the evidence for world-wide Turanian influence is striking, other factors undoubtedly account for similar legends, traditions, and uses for ginseng. For instance, many roots actually do bear some physical resemblance to the human form. Thus, allusion to a "man-image" does not seem surprising.

Botany of the Plant

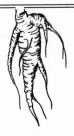

Botany of Ginseng

The ginseng plant belongs to the Araliaciae family. As such, it is closely related to American spikenard (Aralia nudicaulis), Indian spikenard (Aralia racemosa), and, of course, Siberian ginseng (Eleutherococcus senticosus).

Technically, the ginseng plant is a deciduous perennial. In other words, it lives indefinitely for many years, but the foliage dies back at the end of each season. It is not known just how long the ginseng plant can survive, but it probably gets to be an extremely old plant if its growth is undisturbed. Most wild ginseng roots weigh about an ounce, but specimens have been found in Siberia that weigh over ten ounces. Judging from the number of transverse "rings" and bud scars, it would appear that some of these specimens might be as old as 400 years.

Ginseng usually germinates in early spring after a long dormancy period. In the first season, the plant can scarcely be seen even at close range. It bears two or three very small leaves that never reach more than about two inches in height. Each successive year, the plant produces increasingly larger leafstalks, until they reach about a foot in height.

ginseng plant with fruit structure

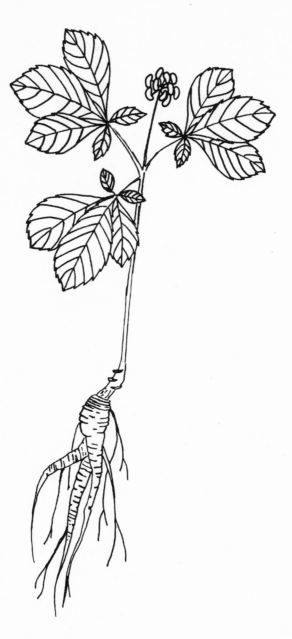

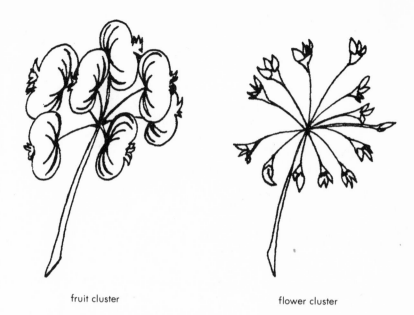

fruit cluster   flower cluster

Every autumn, the leafstalk dies back to the root, where a permanent scar is left on the *neck* (the structure between the root itself and the base of the stem). Simultaneously, the root shrinks slightly into the ground.

Usually, no flowers are produced until the third or fourth year. The flower stalk originates at the point where the leaves come together at the apex of the stalk. The flowers are pale green in color, and they occur in a round cluster known as an umbel. The seeds are soon produced, enclosed in bright red berries. Usually, many more berries are produced by cultivated ginseng than by the wild plant. The berries are edible, as evidenced by the fact that birds and field mice love to eat them. They taste very much like the root, but are considered to have no medicinal properties whatsoever.

The ginseng plant reproduces itself in nature by seed only. The plants usually grow very sparsely, seldom in groups. In the Orient, however, groups of 100 or more plants have been found on rare occasions.

11

Botanical Variation In Ginseng

In recent times, much interbreeding has taken place in the cultivation of ginseng. Consequently, there are few truly pure varieties any more. Many growers of ginseng simply select seeds from what appear to be the healthiest plants in order to start their next crop. Nevertheless, some pure strains of ginseng have been maintained, particularly in the Orient. The following list summarizes these different varieties.

Botanical Name	Characteristics
Panax quinquefolium (regular)	peduncle extends slightly above the petioles; papery scale at base of annual shoot; short, straight root
Panax quinquefolium ("peanut" variety)	peduncle extends slightly above the petioles; papery scale at base of annual shoot; short, crooked root
Panax schinseng (regular)	peduncle extends far beyond the petioles; fleshy scale at base of annual shoot; short, straight root
Panax schinseng ("repens" variety)	peduncle extends far beyond the petioles; fleshy scale at base of annual shoot; long, straight, horizontal root
Panax schinseng ("kamsan" variety)	peduncle extends far beyond the petioles; fleshy scale at base of annual shoot; short, crooked root

Explanation of terms:

peduncle: the stalk of the flowering structure

petiole: the stalk of the leaf

scale: a small protective structure from
which the main stem emerges. After
the main stem emerges, the
scale remains.

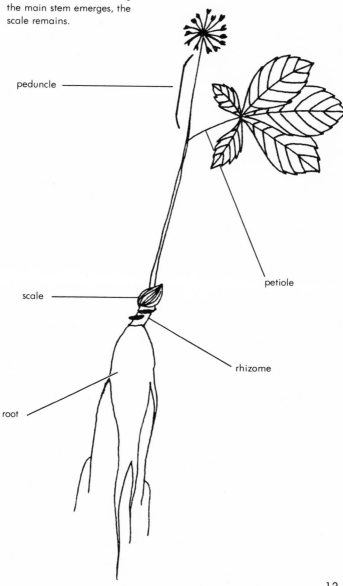

peduncle

petiole

scale

rhizome

root

13

Peculiarities of the Ginseng Plant

One common variation that occurs in ginseng plants is that the plants sometimes produces perfect flowers, and sometimes produce separate staminate and pistillate flowers instead. A plant that has perfect flowers means that the flowers have both stamens and pistils in each flower. (The stamens are the male sexual organs of the flower; the pistils are the female sexual organs of the flower.) A plant that has perfect flowers will produce seed. A plant that has pistillate flowers will produce seed if it is near a staminate plant. A plant that has only staminate flowers cannot produce seed at all. In general, young plants tend to bear perfect flowers; older plants tend to bear staminate or pistillate flowers.

Another rarity in the ginseng plant that is occasionally encountered is the presence of a double embryo seed. One double embryo seed will give rise to two separate plants. This trait is almost never encountered in other members of the plant kingdom.

There is also considerable variation in the appearance of the leaves and roots of ginseng. One variety of *Panax quinquefolium,* known as "peanut ginseng," has small, stubby roots but generally produces an unusually large number of seeds. It was cultivated at one time in the southern United States for its high seed yield.

"peanut" ginseng

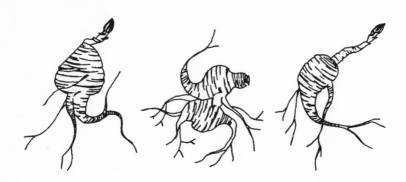

Lastly, it should be mentioned that although ginseng leaflets are ordinarily oblanceolate, strains of ginseng occasionally occur that are exclusively lanceolate.

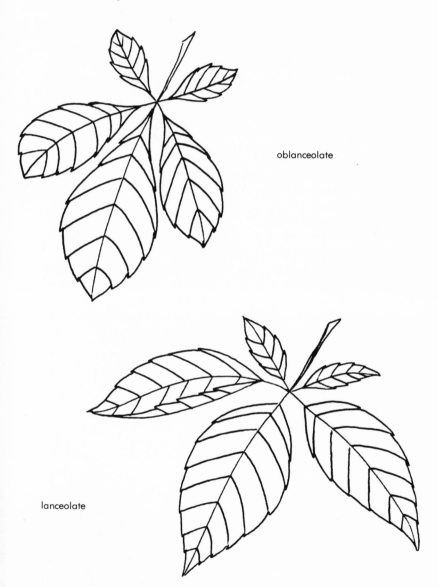

oblanceolate

lanceolate

Contractility of Ginseng

One rather interesting finding that has resulted from recent Soviet studies of ginseng is that the root of the plant contracts just enough each year to perfectly balance the upward growth of the plant. In this way, the bud that appears each spring is situated exactly at the surface level of the ground.

If the root did not contract, the neck of the plant (the area between the root and the bud) would continue to grow further and further above the ground until it collapsed from the weight of the leafy stalk, or until it was broken by falling debris or stepped on by an animal.

Each year after the leafy stalk dies, another scar is left on the neck of the plant. Only one scar is left each year. On the basis of the number of rings that appear on the root (which are caused by annual shrinkage), and on the basis of the number of bud scars that appear on the neck, it is often possible to closely estimate the age of a particular plant. Using this method, a few specimens have been found to be almost half a century old. This method of determining the age of ginseng has been practiced by the Chinese since antiquity, but only recently has scientific investigation confirmed the validity of this method.

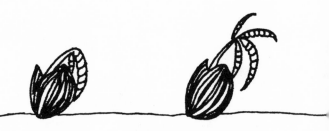

The annual emergence of the leafy stem from the ginseng root. Note the slow unfurling of the leaves and the slight downward recession of the scale.

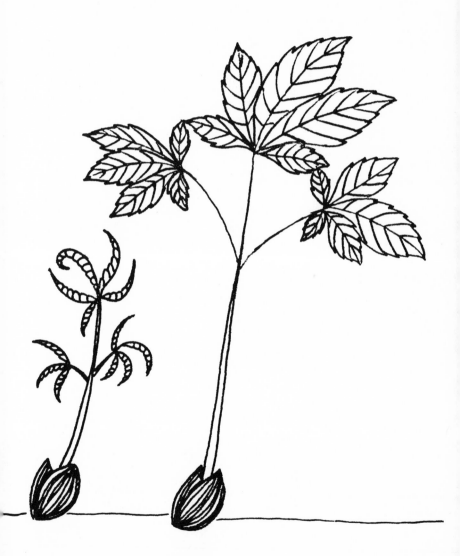

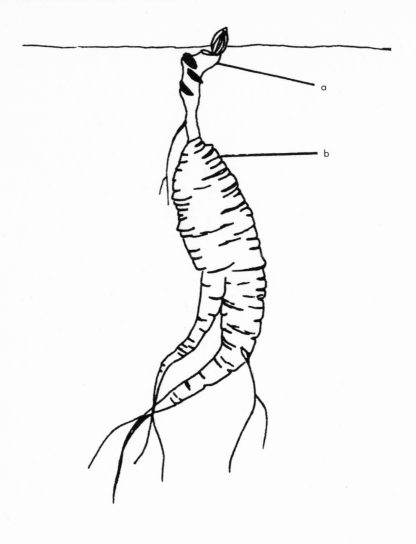

area at (a) grows upward at exactly
the same rate that area at (b) shrinks
downward, so that the top bud is always
exactly at the ground surface level

As a rule, the more "rings" a ginseng root has, the more valuable it is. When the root appears to have many rings, this is believed to be a good indication that the root is also very old, and the older roots command higher prices.

Unfortunately, some unscrupulous merchants have been known to take fresh, young roots and wrap thread around the upper end. The roots are then heated with steam, causing the root to expand and the thread to cut grooves into the root which are sometimes mistaken for rings. Fortunately, however, it is a fairly simple matter to detect this form of fraud. The genuine rings have a quite different appearance. The following chart should clarify the difference:

Genuine Rings

1. The genuine rings are not in the form of perfect circles, but usually follow a wavy pattern.

2. The genuine rings are not continuous, but frequently go part of the way around the root, and then stop.

3. The genuine rings are few in number unless the root is especially large.

4. The genuine rings never follow a spiral formation.

Thread Marks

1. The rings made by thread usually form perfect circles around the root.

2. The fake rings are always continuous, unbroken circles that go all the way around the root.

3. It is not uncommon to find many fake rings on a very small root.

4. The fake rings often follow a spiral formation that can be followed with the fingernail just as the spiral grooves in a screw can be followed.

It should be noted that this tactic is almost never seen on ginseng roots in the United States, but almost exclusively in the Orient (where it is nevertheless a rare practice). In the United States, roots are not usually purchased on the basis of the number of rings, because few Americans realize the significance of these rings.

History of Ginseng

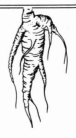

History of Ginseng

One of the earliest literary references to ginseng is found in the *Pen-ts'ao (Herbal)*, which first appeared in written form in China in the first century B.C. An oral tradition relating to ginseng undoubtedly goes back many millenia. Ginseng was also mentioned in the ancient *Atherva Veda* of India, which alludes to its aphrodisiac properties.

At an unknown time in the distant past, there arose a dedicated society of ginseng prospectors known as the *va-pang-suis*. The group consisted of a highly restrictive membership. Only Chinese men of impeccable character could join the *va-pang-suis*. Also, each member had to be capable of enduring the many hazards of this arduous profession. Often they remained for many long weeks in the mountains of northern China and southeastern Russia, far from any outposts of civilization. They were often menaced by the Far Eastern tiger, other wild animals, and numerous vandals who confined their activities exclusively to exploiting and robbing the *va-pang-suis*. Often, even the best prospectors would return with not a single find to show for their hardships in the wilderness. Even those who did manage to find a specimen of wild ginseng seldom obtained more than a tiny fraction of its value.

When the wild roots were brought down from the mountains, they were sold to Chinese pharmacists, who in turn sold them (intact or made into a tincture) to the wealthy Chinese upper class. The wealthy Chinese used ginseng daily; not only as a medicine, but as a condiment and seasoning for many culinary dishes. The poorer Chinese could not use ginseng regularly or even frequently; nevertheless, their faith in ginseng was such that they would often spend their last few cents on the highest grade of ginseng they could buy for the benefit of an ill family member.

At a remote time in history, the Chinese emperors (who used ginseng regularly in large quantities) began to cultivate choice specimens of the finest roots. This gave rise to the famous *mandarin* (imperial) grade of ginseng. For centuries, the imperial crop was improved through a system of hybridization. The largest, strongest, and hardiest plants were interbred, resulting in an excellent strain of cultivated ginseng. *Mandarin* ginseng was used only by the emperor, his family, and his close friends and associates. Occasionally, when an unusually large harvest left an excess of ginseng, the remainder was sold to buyers at enormous prices. Mr. I. F. Shephard, writing in the *United States Consular Reports* (No. 46, vol. XIV, 1884), describes the situation:

> 'Imperial ginseng,' so called because it is raised or gathered under imperial protection in the parks or hunting grounds, where it is kept free from the profanation of the vulgar herd. This variety ranges from $40 to $200 per pound, and is largely taken up by the wealthy classes in Peking and vicinity, as far as I can learn. It is fine in its appearance, quite in the desired form, and of course very scarce in trade.

Around the mid-1700s, the Chinese emperor began a system of licensing ginseng hunters. These "diggers" were given a monetary loan with which to purchase supplies to last through a season spent hunting ginseng in the wilderness. They were also subsidized to hire four assistants. When the season was over, the diggers had to pay back the loan and present the emperor with two ounces of their best finds. The remaining amount was purchased by the emperor. Father Jartoux describes the system:

> These herbarists carry with them neither tents nor beds, everyone being sufficiently loaded with his provision, which is

only millet parched in an oven. So that they are constrained to sleep under trees, having only their branches and barks, if they can find them, for their covering. Each collector should give His Majesty two ounces of the best, and the rest should be paid for according to its weight in fine silver. It was computed that by this means the emperor would get this year, 1709, about 20,000 pounds of it, which would not cost him above one-fourth of its value.

In 1714, Father Jartoux, a missionary for many years among the Chinese, wrote *A Description of a Tartarian Plant Called Ginseng*. In this work, he described the very great esteem in which the Chinese hold ginseng, and described his own personal experiences with it. Having become severely fatigued on one of his voyages through China, he was presented with a small amount of ginseng to chew. After taking the ginseng, his fatigue vanished entirely in less than an hour. Father Jartoux was actually able to correctly predict the discovery of ginseng in North America, based upon a comparison of the climates of China and Canada:

> If it is to be found in any other country in the world, it may be particularly in Canada, where the forests and the mountains, according to the relation of those that have lived there, very much resemble those here (in China).

Father Lafitau, a missonary in Canada, came across the writings of Father Jartoux.

> It was by accident that I first learned of ginseng. I had stopped in Quebec on business connected with out mission in the month of October, 1715. They have a custom of sending us every year a copy of the edifying letters of the missionaries of our company who labor in every part of the world . . . The tenth parcel of these letters fell into my hands, and I read with pleasure one from Father Jartoux. In it I found an exact description of the ginseng plant. . . .

After considerable searching, Father Lafitau found wild ginseng near Montreal:

> . . . in looking for the ginseng, by accident I found it, when I was not thinking of it, near a house I was having built . . . It

was then ripe, and the color of the fruit attracted my attention. I pulled it up, and with joy took it to an Indian I had engaged to help me hunt for it. She recognized it at once as one of those the Indians used.

In a short time, a huge trade had begun. The exportation of American ginseng to the Orient has continued up to the present time. Today, most of the ginseng exported to the Orient from North America is cultivated ginseng, due to the scarcity of the wild variety.

Peter Kalm, a Swedish explorer who traveled through Canada in 1749, gave an early account of the prosperous North American ginseng trade. His travels were recounted in *Voyages and Travels* by John Pinkerton, a monumental geographic anthology published in England in 1812. In the following passage, Kalm alludes to the enormous popularity of North American ginseng in China. The period he refers to would have occured after the discovery of North American ginseng in 1716, but prior to 1752 when a shipment of spoiled ginseng roots to the Orient shattered the faith of the Oriental buyers for many years. In fact, it took about a century for the market to fully recover.

> The French use this root for curing the asthma, as a stomachic, and to promote fertility in women. The trade which is carried on with it here is brisk; for they gather great quantities of it, and send them to France, from whence they are brought to China, and sold there to great advantage . . . During my stay in Canada, all the merchants at Quebec and Montreal received orders from their correspondents in France to send over a quantity of ginseng, there being an uncommon demand for it in this summer. The roots were accordingly collected in Canada with all possible diligence; the Indians especially traveled about the country in order to collect as much as they could, and to sell it to the merchants at Montreal. The Indians in the neighborhood of this town were likewise so much taken up with this business that the French farmers were not able during that time to hire a single Indian, as they commonly do, to help in the harvest. Many people feared lest by continuing for several successive years to collect these plants without leaving one or two in each place to propagate their species, there

A

GENERAL COLLECTION

OF THE

BEST AND MOST INTERESTING

VOYAGES AND TRAVELS

IN ALL PARTS OF THE WORLD;

MANY OF WHICH ARE NOW FIRST TRANSLATED INTO ENGLISH.

DIGESTED ON A NEW PLAN.

BY JOHN PINKERTON,

AUTHOR OF MODERN GEOGRAPHY, &c. &c.

ILLUSTRATED WITH PLATES.

VOLUME THE THIRTEENTH.

LONDON:

PRINTED FOR LONGMAN, HURST, REES, ORME, AND BROWN, PATERNOSTER-ROW ;
AND CADELL AND DAVIES, IN THE STRAND.

1812.

would soon be very few of them left, which I think is very likely to happen, for by all accounts they formerly grew in abundance round Montreal; but at present there is not a single plant of it to be found, so effectually have they been rooted up. This obliged the Indians, this summer, to go far within the English boundaries to collect these roots.

Ginseng and the New England Colonists

William E. Griffis, writing in the late nineteenth century, gives a very informative account of the role of ginseng in the commerce of the New England colonies around the time of the American Revolutionary War.

At a rather early date, the Dutch settlers in New York heard about the discovery of ginseng in Canada. This event stimulated a thorough search of their colonial territory for the ginseng plant. The search ended in the discovery of ginseng near Stockbridge, Massachusetts. The Indians native to this region quickly learned that they could trade the roots with the Dutch merchants in Albany in exchange for hardware, trinkets, and rum. The Dutch merchants, in turn, sold the roots to the Chinese at an enormous profit. It is interesting to note that a famous Puritan of the time, Jonathan Edwards, was quick to condemn the Indians for the "debauchery" that supposedly ensued in exchanging the ginseng for rum. Perhaps this is not so much a reflection on the behavior of the Indians as on Edwards' total intolerance of liquor.

It was not long before larger and larger amounts of ginseng were shipped from the New England colonies to the Orient, while considerable quantities of tea were being shipped from the Orient to the New England colonies.

The colonists in the New World, however, did not make the profit from the sale of this ginseng, and were unjustly taxed for the tea. The profit, instead, was going to the European nations that owned the colonies. Many colonists felt that they had to endure the hardships of living in the New World. Why, then, should England and Holland have the right to sell their native resources and control their foreign trade? Also, why should they be forced to pay taxes on imports such as tea?

This was one of the causes of resentment between the colonists and their distant European rulers that eventually led to the Boston Tea Party and, finally, the American Revolution. A patriotic colonial spokesman had this in mind when he said:

> the Americans must have tea, and they seek the most lucrative market for their precious root ginseng.

> —Captain Samuel Shaw,
> first U.S. consul to China.

Even George Washington mentioned ginseng in his diary after a visit to Ohio in 1784:

> In passing over the mountains, I met numbers of persons and pack horses going in with ginseng.

Daniel Boone, however, was not content to simply write about ginseng. He gathered the roots in Kentucky in 1788 and shipped them up the Ohio River from whence they were sent to Philadelphia.

The Eradication of Oriental Wild Ginseng

Over the centuries, the supply of wild ginseng in Asia has gradually dwindled to almost nothing. Today, it can only be found in the Sikhote-Alin Mountains of Siberia, and in parts of Korea and Manchuria. But even in these regions it is extremely rare and almost extinct. The following is a summary of the events that led to the current short supply of wild Asiatic ginseng.

In summary, wild Asiatic ginseng may have once grown in Nepal near India's northern border, and in central China through Manchuria, northern Korea, and into far-eastern Russia. Today, it is found almost exclusively in the Sikhote-Alin Mountains of the far-eastern USSR.

It should be noted, however, that most of the areas in which Asiatic ginseng once grew wild are now areas in which ginseng is cultivated to some extent.

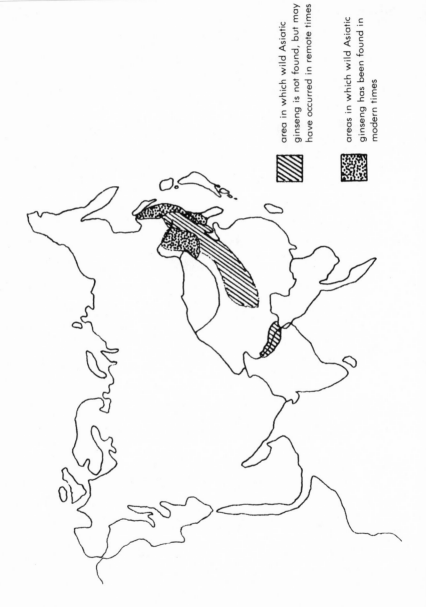

area in which wild Asiatic ginseng is not found, but may have occurred in remote times

areas in which wild Asiatic ginseng has been found in modern times

28

Events

Period	Events
Han Dynasties (202 B.C.–220 A.D.)	The *Pen-ts'ao (Herbal)* first appears in written form in China. This marks one of the earliest literary references to ginseng.
Northern Dynasties (386–581 A.D.)	Hung-king wrote on Korean ginseng, stating that ginseng and the kia tree have "mutual sympathy." For this reason, he said, ginseng is often found growing in the shade of the kia tree.
Ming Dynasty (1368–1644)	The consumption of ginseng in China increases. The supply in the T'ai-hang Mountains of Shansi is exhausted; Liao-tung, Korea, and Chien-chou Juchen become new sources.
Manchu Dynasty (1644–1912)	The ginseng trade falls under strict governmental control. The government issues special licenses which permit digging in Sheng-ching. Later, the government digging grounds are extended to include northern Manchuria. Soon, ginseng found in Ninguta and Ula near Kirin is exploited almost to the point of extinction. Diggers then turned to the Heje and Ussuri regions.
Republic (1912–1949)) and People's Republic of China (1949–present)	Wild Asiatic ginseng is found almost exclusively in the Sikhote-Alin Mountains of the Ussuri region of the U.S.S.R. On rare occasions, a wild specimen is discovered in Manchuria or northern Korea.

Dersu the Trapper

The late V. K. Arseniev, a Russian, spent much time in the exploration of Siberia at the beginning of the twentieth century. During his travels, he made the acquaintance of Dersu Uzala, trapper and hunter of ginseng. (In Asia and in North America, trappers often work in the areas where wild ginseng grows; consequently, they keep an eye open for the plant. For this reason, many companies that deal in the fur trade in North America also deal in ginseng as a sideline.) Dersu and Arseniev became very good friends, and Arseniev was able to learn a great deal about ginseng from Dersu. He relates his adventures in his book, *Dersu the Trapper*. The book was translated from the Russian in 1939, and makes for excellent reading, especially for anyone interested in ginseng.

Arseniev described the existence of ginseng plantations in the Sikhote-Alin region, which had previously been unknown to the outside world. He also gave clear and detailed descriptions of the ginseng prospector and his ways. He describes their simple clothing and the small, portable huts in which they live alone for weeks in the wilderness. The ginseng hunter lives in the wilderness with a few simple tools essential to his work—a knife, a piece of bone for digging ginseng roots, some primitive spades, rakes, and shovels, and a few birch boxes of variable sizes.

An Early Siberian Account

E. G. Ravenstein, in *The Russians On the Amur* (1861), quotes from the writings of de la Bruniere, an early French explorer of the Sikhote-Alin region of Russia. De la Bruniere describes the Chinese ginseng hunters in that region in grimly pessimistic terms:

> These men, wretched in their entire being, have here no other means of sustaining life than that of giving themselves up, with incredible fatigue, to the search of the ginseng. Picture to yourself one of these miserable carriers, laden with more than twenty-four pounds weight, venturing without any road across immense forests, climbing up or descending the mountains; always left alone to his own thoughts, and exposed to every distemper; not knowing if today or tomorrow he may fall a victim to the wild beasts which abound around him, supported

THE

RUSSIANS ON THE AMUR;

ITS

DISCOVERY, CONQUEST, AND COLONISATION,

WITH

A DESCRIPTION OF THE COUNTRY, ITS INHABITANTS, PRODUCTIONS, AND COMMERCIAL CAPABILITIES;

AND

PERSONAL ACCOUNTS OF RUSSIAN TRAVELLERS.

BY

E. G. RAVENSTEIN, F.R.G.S.

CORRESPONDING FELLOW OF THE GEOGRAPHICAL SOCIETY OF FRANKFURT

ILLUSTRATED BY

Three Maps, Four Plates & Fifty-Eight Wood Engravings.

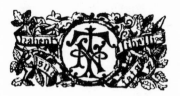

LONDON:

TRUBNER AND CO., PATERNOSTER ROW.

—

1861.

31

by the modicum of millet he brings with him, and a few wild herbs to season it. And all this during five months of the year, from the end of April to the end of September.

In a later section, he describes a ginseng plantation:

On the 17th of July we come to the mouth of the Vongo; the Usuri here flows between the mountains. We found a ginseng plantation, and inquired into the cultivation of this plant. The settlement numbers twenty hands, all of them Chinese, and belongs to a rich merchant who lives at Peking. Considering the value of this plant in China, the proprietor of these few acres must draw from them an immense revenue. More than thirty beds, each about thirty-five yards long, and four feet wide, are planted in rows with this expensive root. The berries were not yet ripe, but had begun to get red. The beds are protected against the sun by tents or by sheds of wood. The earth must be a rich black mould and loose. When the plant has attained a height of four or five inches it is supported by a stick. The beds are carefully weeded and watered. The plantation is surrounded by a hedge and carefully guarded. The guard is strictly forbidden to sell any root, and our endeavors to purchase one were in vain.

He probably feared the other laborers might betray him to the proprietors, but when we left he invited us to pay him a visit on our return, and gave us to understand that then he might possibly gratify our wish. I heard that there were many such plantations in the neighborhood, and was anxious to know where, and at what prices the root was sold. The Chinese themselves answered evasively or not at all, but our guide told us they were taken to Hun-chun and there sold to merchants who either carried them across the sea or inland.

Packaging of Ginseng

Great care is always taken in the packing and storing of high-grade ginseng. Normally, the roots are stored in wooden boxes with glass lids. If there are many tiny rootlets present, they are padded with ample cotton-wool to prevent their breakage. An early account of 1895 describes some of the methods then in use:

The greatest care is taken of the pieces of finest quality. M. Huc says that throughout China no chemist's shop is unprovided with more or less of it. According to the account given by Lockhart *(Medical Missionary in China)* of a visit to a ginseng merchant, it is stored in boxes lined with sheet lead, which are kept in larger boxes containing quicklime for absorbing moisture. The pieces of the precious drug are further enclosed in silk wrappers and kept in little silk-lined boxes. The merchant, when showing a piece bared of wrappings to Mr. Lockhart for his inspection, requested him not to breathe on or handle it, while he dilated on its merits, and related the marvelous cures he had known it to effect. The root is covered, according to quality, with the finest embroidered silk, plain cotton cloth, or paper."

In other accounts, reference is made to wrapping the roots in tin foil by the *va-pang-suis.* It was believed that handling a root not covered by the foil could result in a peculiar sort of "ginseng sickness."

At the present time, the custom of wrapping ginseng in tin foil or lead foil remains a mystery. Some writers have speculated that the root, which they say prefers radioactive soil, accumulates radiation and can emit this radiation in dangerous amounts if a person receives too much exposure to it.

Actually, there is little scientific evidence that ginseng *prefers* radioactive soil. However, many plants are capable of *storing* radiation in dangerous amounts *if* they are exposed to it.

The Chemulpho Customs Incident

For many years, the export of Korean red ginseng was totally forbidden in all treaties made between Korea and the outside world. Korean white ginseng was, however, one of Korea's major exports.

During the latter part of the nineteenth century, the demand for red ginseng in China greatly exceeded the supply. The Chinese sought to import red ginseng from neighboring Korea, but they were refused on several occasions. Tension between the two countries grew steadily worse, and smuggling was not uncommon. Then, in January 1886, a major incident occured between the Korean customs officers at Chemulpho and the Chinese local residents. The following account of the incident by George C. Foulk of the U.S. Navy, appeared in *Foreign Relations of the United States* for 1886. It is an excellent illustration of the tremendous value placed on red ginseng by the Chinese, who had become desperate to obtain it after numerous attempts to obtain Korean red ginseng by legitimate means:

It appears that some time since the customs officers at Chemulpho received word that a discharged telegraph operator, a Chinese, was buying up quantities of red ginseng in Corea; and again they learned recently that a large quantity of red ginseng was about to be sent from Seoul to Chemulpho. In anticipation of an attempt of the Chinese to smuggle this red ginseng out of Corea through Chemulpho, they increased their watchfulness, and it would appear that by the 25th ultimo every avenue of escape of the ginseng had been closed at Chemulpho.

For several days before the 25th, parties of Chinese had been coming down from Seoul, many of them to take passage for China aboard the Chinese gunboat Ching Hai, which was to sail on the morning of the 26th. These civilian passengers were furnished with passes to go in the gunboat by the Chinese consul at Chemulpho. Among them was one Ling, who was suspected of being the leader in the case of ginseng smuggling at hand. . . . In all, upwards of twenty Chinese subjects were to take passage on the gunboat.

On the afternoon of January 25th the commissioner of customs at the Chemulpho consul went to the Chinese consul there to confer with him in regard to the right of the customs officers to make search of effects of persons to sail in the Chinese gunboat, such search having been protested against by the Chinese on various grounds, chief of which was that they had passes from the Chinese authorities to take passage in her, and she was a Chinese naval vessel. While this conference was in progress one of the customs officers learned that a large quantity of ginseng had already been placed on board the gunboat, and that a further quantity was to go on during the evening. A little later, about 5 p.m., he heard that a determined attempt—to involve fighting if necessary—would be made by the Chinese in combination that evening to get their ginseng off to the gunboat.

At about 7 o'clock, a Chinese was stopped at the custom house on his way to the beach, by a Corean watchman, whom the

Chinaman promptly struck. An American of the customs service, Mr. Charles Welch, went to the rescue of the watchman, and led the Chinaman to the general office, to retain him there until the commissioner returned. The Chinaman called out for assistance, and was heard over the Chinese settlement, which is close by. In a few minutes Mr. Welch was set upon by eight or nine Chinese, the leader being Ling. He was cuffed and beaten, but escaped without serious injury.

At the same time the customs offices were filled with the Chinese who were in the settlement, whose manner was threatening and excited. A secretary of the consul, who was present, warned the customs officers, most of whom were foreigners, to escape from the offices, as an attack was about to be made. They had hardly gotten clear of the rooms when the mob began to demolish the furniture. The windows were smashed, and the room and part of the building made a wreck. The customs officers having been driven away, the custom house was left in possession of the Chinese, with a clear field to dispose of their effects as they willed. The Chinese consul appeared later on the scene, and summoned twelve sailors from a Chinese gunboat in the harbor. The Chinese mob then dispersed, and the Chinese sailors remained to guard the custom-house during the night, with several of the customs officers who had returned to their post.

On the following morning the entire Chinese community united in a demonstration against the customs foreign employees, which was shown by their closing their places of business, one of which is a hotel at which the customs officers take their meals. The English vice-consul vigorously enjoined the Chinese consul to take steps to suppress the disorder, and the latter issued a proclamation, a copy of translation of which I enclose. In this the people were directed to open their shops, which was done. On the morning of the 26th the guard of sailors was relieved at the custom house by one of Chinese marines.

It would appear that on the morning of the 26th, Ling, with others of the Chinese who had come from Seoul, was actively engaged in fomenting further trouble. . . . At about 11 a.m. a party of the riotous Chinese went in search of a Corean customs watchman, and utterly destroyed a watch-house on the beach.

As there was every appearance of further trouble, in case of which it was believed the Chinese guard of marines would be useless or inefficient, Mr. Stripling (English), the commissioner of customs, urgently requested of Mr. Parker the use of a guard of English marines from the Swift, then lying in port, to protect the customs. Acceding to this, the English marines were summoned by Mr. Parker rather for the protection of the English consulate. They had not yet arrived, when the Chinese again closed their shops and gathered in a threatening body at the customs house, the Seoul Chinese being the leaders. At this time a serious affray was only prevented by the endeavors of the customs officers to prevent the Chinese marines from firing into the mob. At the most critical time the English marines approached on their way from the Swift. This had the effect of quieting the mob, which slowly dispersed.

With this the affair was practically ended, though many threatening rumors were current for several days.

The gravity of the affair as a lawless demonstration, involving acts of violence on the part of a community of Chinese subjects against an institution of Corea, was fully brought to the notice of the Chinese authorities at Chemulpho and in Seoul by the foreign representatives.

The Chinese consul at Chemulpho was summoned to Seoul, and brought with him a number of the riotous Chinese. Mr. Yuen at once began a trial, which was attended by Mr. Merrill, the chief commissioner of customs of Corea, and Mr. Welch, the customs officer who had been assaulted. After a few hours' deliberation Mr. Yuen, the Chinese representative in Seoul, announced the trial ended, and that four Chinese were convicted and would be severely beaten, and deported. These Chinese had taken a wholly insignificant part in the affair, while the head, Ling, and other leaders in the affair, had been exempted from punishment. During the trial so marked a disposition of the Chinese court to screen these leaders was shown, that Mr. Merrill despaired of obtaining justice and left the court, and telegraphed an appeal to the viceroy, Li Hung Chang.

This appeal would appear to have been effective, for on the following day a rehearing of the case was held by Mr. Yuen, from which resulted the conviction of the six principal actors in the affair, including Ling, and their sentence of deportation from Corea; while an order was issued to cause the Chinese community at Chemulpho to make good the damage committed on the customs-house. It was shown conclusively that the customs officers had simply done their duty and were clear from any charge whatsoever against them.

After the first hearing of this case by Mr. Yuen, the president of the foreign office ordered a Corean watchman of the customs to be severely punished, doubtlessly at the instance of Mr. Yuen. Mr. Merrill vigorously protested against this, and caused the order to be revoked. . . .

This outrage upon the Corean customs partakes strongly of the character of a strong protest on the part of the Chinese community in Corea against their being required to pay duties to Corea or subject themselves to the customs laws in other respects. . . .

The recent disturbance at Chemulpho, as based upon attempts to smuggle red ginseng, has already given rise to discussion as to the expediency of making new regulations relative to the red ginseng export from Corea. At present the export is wholly forbidden under the treaties, and the whole crop of red ginseng is carried to China by the annual Corean embassy overland, the greater part to be sold in Peking. Ginseng can only be cured to become "red ginseng" by the agents of His Majesty the King of Corea at Songto. A part of the crop is given to the embassy to China as compensation for services; the balance is the exclusive property of the King. The whole crop is estimated at about 1,000 piculs, the highest estimate of revenue being $240,000. A tax is collected on the ginseng farms at Songto and on the ginseng in transit to China at Oiju, the aggregate of these taxes being commonly reported as sufficient to meet half the expenses of the government. Ginseng has a fabulous value as a medicine to the Chinese, and attempts to smuggle it are only to be expected. The difficulties of preventing this, under the present system of management of the crop, would seem to be almost insurmountable. It has been proposed that the export of it be permitted at the open ports under high duties.

George C. Foulk
Ensign, U.S. Navy

Ginseng Legends

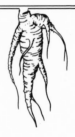

The Man-Image

In reference to ginseng, a *man-image* is a ginseng root that resembles the human figure to a significant degree. The greater the resemblance to the human form, the more valuable the root. If the two lower extremities or *legs* are of equal length, the root is considered to be male. If the two "legs" are of unequal length, the root is considered female. In Chinese tradition, the male form is regarded as slightly more perfect and desirable than the female form. This is apparently a manifestation of a cultural bias, rather than a supportable observation.

A *man-image* root is all the more valuable if it has been found in the wild state. However, Asiatic wild ginseng is always far more valuable than wild North American ginseng, regardless of the appearance of the root.

Another factor that influences the value of a *man-image* is the age of the root. The older roots are the most valuable. An older root can be easily identified from its greater size and weight, the presence of rings near the top of the root, and the number of bud scars on the rhizome.

Finally, it is very important that all of the rootlets are intact, even the tiniest ones. The ginseng hunters of Asia have developed an

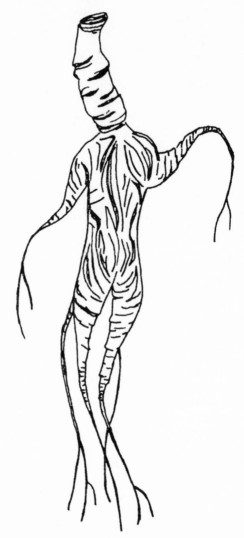

Manchurian wild ginseng: a rare, priceless specimen

interesting method of accomplishing this. They look for a nearby stream, and then carefully channel the water over the root they wish to unearth. The running water slowly washes away the soil, leaving every rootlet perfectly intact. After the root is unearthed, it is then even more difficult to preserve the tiny rootlets because they are very brittle after the root has been dried. (They are fairly resilient while the root is still fresh.) To preserve the tiny rootlets after the ginseng root has been unearthed, one of two methods is used. Either the root is very carefully placed in a sturdy wooden box generously padded with cotton, or the root is placed in a thick glass cylindrical container, and preserved in a strongly alcoholic solution. With the latter method, the alcoholic solution can later be used as a powerful ginseng extract.

If the *man-image* meets all of the above requirements, it is extremely rare and immensely valuable. It may even become legendary. One such root, on display at a permanent exhibit in Moscow, is said to be insured for about $25,000. Others have been bought and sold for many thousands of dollars.

Ginseng Street

Parts of Shanghai are divided into separate districts, each district specializing in one type of merchandise. In addition to such areas as "Sandalwood Street," and "Coffin Street," there is also "Ginseng Street," in which most of the ginseng dealers are concentrated.

In a very fascinating search, Louise Crane wrote on how she spoke to the various merchants of Ginseng Street, trying to learn more about the highest grades of Manchurian wild ginseng. Many of the merchants admitted to having witnessed transactions in which exceptional roots were bought and sold for thousands of dollars, but none of the merchants admitted to having been involved personally in any such transaction. None of the merchants had a genuine Manchurian wild ginseng specimen to show her.

After much searching, one merchant showed Louise Crane a photograph of a root that may have been worth as much as ten thousand dollars. Louise Crane offered to buy the picture; but the merchant vehemently refused to sell it at any price, declaring the *photograph itself* "priceless." Apparently, the other merchants she encountered in her tour displayed an attitude of secrecy, even distrust. Admittedly, the merchants may have had good cause to behave in this manner. After all, if you or I owned a priceless gem, would we be willing to show it to a stranger who came to the door asking about it?

On the basis of this and other bits of information, it is my opinion that high quality Oriental wild ginseng is certainly never displayed in shops, and never finds its way to the Occident at all. We may find good to excellent ginseng offered for sale by herb dealers; but this is the ginseng of commerce. The best specimens of Oriental wild ginseng are analogous to legendary jewels such as the Star of India or the Hope Diamond. If displayed at all, the most elaborate security precautions are taken. They seldom, if ever, change hands.

The Va-pang-suis

Partly because of the decline of the wealthy class of Chinese subsequent to the communist revolution in China, and partly because of the growing scarcity of the Oriental wild ginseng, there are considerably fewer ginseng prospectors in existence today than in the past.

Ginseng hunting was the profession of the *va-pang-suis,* and it was apparently an extremely dangerous activity that would not have been done were it not for the generous sums of money that wealthy Chinese individuals were willing to pay for genuine wild ginseng.

One of the primary hazards of ginseng prospecting was the danger of an encounter with the numerous bandits who sought the prospectors who had found ginseng, or knew where to look for it. These bandits, known as the "White Swans," thought nothing of murdering the *va-pang-suis* and stealing their finds, or of torturing them in order to learn the location of some wild ginseng plants.

There are many other legends regarding the perils of ginseng prospecting. In *Man and Mystery in Asia,* Mr. Ferdinand Ossendowski relates an encounter with a Chinese ginseng prospector in the Sikhote-Alin Mountains, believed to be the source of the most potent wild ginseng in the world. The old prospector tells of tigers and panthers that also hunt the root, and who will kill any human in order to take the root for themselves. He further states that the greatest peril of all is the existence of a small, fiery spirit that guards the root and has supposedly brought many hunters to their deaths. It is said that the small demon can assume the form of the ginseng plant itself, and appear to retreat further and further from the hunter, until he has traveled too far into the forest to ever again find his way to safety.

The *va-pang-suis* were very sincere in their belief that the predators of the forest (animal and human) could never harm a man who was truly pure of heart. Rather than carry weapons, they worshipped the spirits of the forest, the spirits of the tiger, and the panther, and, especially, the great Spirit of the Mountain. They believe that the wild animals of the forest are destined to guard the ginseng, but will only guard it against evil men.

They enter the forest, armed only with a stick. As might be expected, they frequently were robbed by the vandals who prey on the ginseng prospectors. The vandals had a strange custom of presenting their victims with a red-bordered flag, so that other robbers would know that they had already been victimized and would not bother them. Part of the peculiar ethical system of these bandits included a belief that no prospector should be robbed twice in one journey!

When a prospector finds a root, he interprets this as proof that he is actually pure of heart. He assembles an altar of branches, recites various prayers, and then meticulously unearths the root, taking care to leave even the tiniest rootlets intact. He then places the root in a special wooden box, hides it on his person, and proceeds back to the town pretending as though he had found nothing until he reaches the merchant to whom he will sell it.

The true prospector, whether he has found many roots or no roots at all, will faithfully return every year into the forest to seek for the plant.

The Doctrine of Signatures

Among the legends that concern ginseng, one frequently encounters the belief that the part of the root that resembles a part of the human anatomy should be used to treat afflictions in the corresponding area of the body. The *arms* of the roots should be used for arm ailments; the *head* of the root should be used for head ailments, and so on.

This belief is common to many different regions of the world. It can be found among the North American Indians, the Chinese, the Europeans, and others.

In the European tradition, this concept is known as the Doctrine of Signatures. The idea first appeared in the Middle Ages. Advocates of this concept point out that part of the *Bible* (Book of Genesis) in which God gives to man "every green plant" for his use. It was noted that certain plants have an outward resemblance to a particular part of the body. From this came the conclusion that God gives man a clue as to how each medicinal plant should be used. This clue, or sign, is the plant's signature. Thus, bloodroot (whose root exudes a blood-red liquid) is used to treat certain blood diseases; liverworts (which bear a resemblance to the liver) are used to treat liver ailments; bladderworts (which have tiny air bladders) are used to treat bladder ailments, and so on.

A similar concept also applies to animal substances. For instance, certain primitive cultures ate animal brains to treat brain disorders. Liver is sometimes eaten to treat liver ailments. Both practices are actually somewhat substantiated by modern science. The high concentration of RNA and DNA in brain may have potential uses in treating memory disorders. Liver is very useful in treating a particular kind of anemia in which the patient's liver is unable to manufacture the "intrinsic factor." The intrinsic factor is essential to healthy blood formation. A person suffering from an underactive thyroid gland may be given tablets that are made from desiccated animal thyroids.

From a scientific viewpoint, it is often true that a part of an animal's anatomy can be used to treat an ailment in a corresponding part of the human anatomy. Whether the same thing applies to the use of plants in this manner (Doctrine of Signatures) remains questionable. Actual evidence to support this theory is lacking; but many cultures firmly believe in it. It is possible that there is an element of magic or sorcery involved. In a manner of speaking, the Doctrine of Signatures is the exact reverse of voodoo. For instance, certain practitioners claim to have the power to take a photograph of a sick person and either diagnose or treat the patient by concentrating intensely on the photograph. The patient is thereby treated through an image bearing his resemblance. Similarly, witches can use a wax doll or strand of hair from a victim to cause harm to an individual. Just as voodoo may be explainable in terms of magic, this might also be the key to understanding the Doctrine of Signatures.

A Ginseng Legend

Nearly every plant with any economic significance at all has associated with it a legend as to how the plant came to be. These legends are, for the most part, mostly fictional, but the symbolism is often very interesting. If we could learn to read between the lines of this symbolism, so to speak, we could very probably have a greater insight into the true meaning of the legend.

A very ancient and popular Chinese legend about man's first encounter with the ginseng root is related by Dr. F. Porter Smith in *Chinese Materia Medica:*

> It is related that during the reign of Wenti, of the Sui Dynasty (581 to 601 A.D.), at Shanghai in Shensi, at the back of a certain person's house, was heard each night the imploring voice of a man, and when search was made for the source of this sound, at the distance of about a *li* there was seen a remarkable ginseng plant. Upon digging into the earth to the depth of five feet the root was secured, having the shape of a man, with four extremities perfect and complete; and it was this that had been calling out in the night with a man's voice. It was therefore called *T'u-ching*, 'spirit of the ground.' It is said that the best ginseng formerly came from this Shangtang, but at present no true ginseng is produced in that part of Shansi. . . .

In a legend recounted by Dr. F. Porter Smith in *Chinese Materia Medica*, a sort of "test" is described that is used to authenticate a genuine wild ginseng root:

> It is said that in order to test for true ginseng, two persons walk together, one with a piece of the drug in his mouth and the other with his mouth empty. If at the end of five *li* the one with

> the ginseng in his mouth does not feel himself tired, while the other is out of breath, the drug is true.

Although a *li* can sometimes refer to a unit of weight, it is used here as a unit of distance. Five *li* is approximately two miles.

Father Jartoux, while a missionary in Manchuria, also spoke of the anti-fatigue properties of ginseng:

> . . . a sovereign remedy for all weaknesses occasioned by excessive fatigues either of body or mind.

There are several legends that mention the alleged ability of the ginseng root to leave the ground, and then to assume an animal or human form.

The *va-pang-suis* maintained a belief that the older and stronger roots could assume the form of the Ussuri tiger.

Another ancient Chinese legend states that, after 300 years, the ginseng root can leave the earth in the form of a human being. During the 300 years in which the root remains buried, it assumes a more and more human shape as the years go by. After three centuries have passed, it emerges from the ground. Although the creature appears to be human, it possesses a strange type of blood that is pure white in color. The *va-pang-suis* dream of luring this creature because, they say, if some of its white blood can be obtained, its power is so great that a few drops can restore life to a dead man. It is believed that this creature is extremely evasive, and very difficult to capture.

The legend also states that the strange humanoid creature will soon leave the Earth, and dwell forever among the stars and heavenly bodies.

Many available ginseng preparations bear a symbolic representation of this legend on their labels. A ginseng plant is depicted with its branches reaching up to the sky. The leaves are slightly distorted so that they have the appearance of five-pointed stars that reach into the heavens.

Another very ancient legend is used to explain the origin of ginseng. For a ginseng plant to emerge, a bolt of lightning must first strike a mountain stream. The lightning subsequently leaves a jagged hole in the ground, into which the mountain stream flows. The ginseng plant is formed in the mold left by the lightning bolt. The root of the plant contains and stores the power of the lightning bolt and the power of the flowing water. To possess the ginseng root is to possess these powers. To consume the ginseng root is to unleash these powers within the body. This power, according to the legend, is sufficient to insure health and well-being in anyone.

The Ginseng Mystery

To some observers, it has always seemed strange and inconsistent that $200 an ounce was once the price of the finest imperial ginseng, while American ginseng fell into such unpopularity that it was finally excluded from the *United States Pharmacoepia*.

For centuries, Chinese imperial ginseng was used by the emperor, his family, and his friends, and administered to important government officials (and other important citizens) only when they were deemed to be in such bad health that their usefulness to the emperor was in jeopardy. Many stories have been told about persons who were essentially on their deathbeds, who were restored to health in a very short time following the administration of imperial ginseng.

Actually, a difference in the effects of the various grades of ginseng is entirely feasible. When a botanical drug in one part of the world is also grown at another, distant location, there is apt to be considerable variation in the plant's chemical content.

For example, Chinese *Ephedra (ma-huang)* is many times more potent than the *Ephedra* native to the western United States. In fact, the alkaloid ephedrine is found in very large quantities in the Chinese plant, but the American plant contains little or no ephedrine.

A major difference can also be seen in a comparison of Peruvian coca leaves with Java coca leaves. The Peruvian variety is very rich in the alkaloid cocaine; but the Javanese plant contains primarily ecgonine; but very little cocaine. It is interesting to note that Javanese coca is botanically identical in every way to Peruvian coca, from which it originated.

It is a fact that most of the research that has been done in recent years has used primarily Korean ginseng. Some time ago, the Russians obtained about twenty-two million dollars worth of Korean ginseng. The supply was enough to undertake extensive research on ginseng; and, in fact, the great majority of research on ginseng has been done by the Russians. Chinese, American, and Japanese ginseng has never been adequately studied in controlled experiments. Of course, any study using the higher grades of Chinese ginseng would necessarily be a tremendously expensive project. Chemists and pharmacologists are not able to finance their own research projects; and it would be necessary to apply to an institute or large company for the necessary funds. It is understandable that anyone would hesitate to finance such a costly experiment; but there is much reason to believe that a chemical and/or pharmacological comparison of Chinese imperial ginseng with Korean, American, and Japanese ginseng could potentially contribute a great deal to our knowledge of this intriguing substance.

Ginseng and the Mandrake

Probably no two plants resemble one another more closely with respect to history and folklore than ginseng and the mandrake (*Mandragora officinarum*). Except for the fact that early illustrations appear to represent two different plants, one might otherwise suppose that ginseng and the mandrake are synonymous. The following is a summary of the similar legends surrounding the two plants:

1. Most striking, perhaps, are the stories that allude to roots having a human-like form. In the Orient, ginseng roots that have a humanoid appearance are far more valuable, and very large prices have been paid for such roots. The word "ginseng" actually comes from the Chinese *jen-shen,* meaning "man root." Surprisingly, an American Indian word for the plant, *garantoquen,* means the same.

With respect to the legendary mandrake, root specimens carved into humanoid shapes have been used for centuries throughout the world. Such roots are believed to be extremely potent love charms, capable of producing fertility, warding off illness, and bringing prosperity to the owner. No one knows for certain how the term "mandrake" originated; but in certain languages, the word has obvious allusions to the humanoid appearance of the root. In Persian, for example, mandrake is called *merdomingia,* meaning "man-like plant."

2. There are traditional legends about both ginseng and the mandrake that mention an alleged ability of these plants to glow in the dark. In particular, with respect to the mandrake, the Arabs and the Moors refer to this unusual tendency. It is, however, somewhat feasible, because it is said that in North Africa a certain type of insect, resembling the glowworm, has an affinity for the plant and tends to congregate on the leaves.

There are legends, also, which refer to the ability of the ginseng plant to glow in the dark—but apparently for another reason. It is believed by some that the professional hunters of Oriental wild ginseng, the *va-pang-suis,* are able to find the plants at night by the perception of an unusual glow. It has been proposed that the glow is due to the tendency of ginseng to thrive in radioactive soil; but this has never been proven conclusively.

3. Another interesting way in which the ginseng and the mandrake resemble each other is their traditional use in cases of sterility and impotence, and as an aphrodisiac.

In Chinese medicine, ginseng is considered the supreme remedy for any sort of sexual inadequacy. The very finest grades of Chinese ginseng are reputed to have the power to restore fertility, even to those who have long passed the normal childbearing age. Stories have been told of persons well over the age of 100 who have had children.

Similar stories are told regarding the role of the mandrake as a fertility agent and an aphrodisiac. The ancient Greek writer, Dioscorides, who is generally regarded as the "father of herbalism," mentioned its role as an important ingredient of love philtres. It has long been used in Europe and parts of Asia to induce fertility. For this purpose, it is either taken internally or worn as an amulet. A common English synonym for mandrake, "love apple," is derived from the traditional use of the plant as an aphrodisiac.

Grades of Ginseng

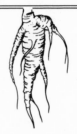

Grades of Ginseng

Ginseng varies considerably in size, shape, color, form, and so on. Consequently, there are many different grades of ginseng. Depending upon its quality, ginseng can vary in price from about $3 per ounce to as much as $100 per ounce. In actuality, the very finest grades of ginseng seldom, if ever, leave the Orient at all. Thus, the ginseng available in the United States never really approaches $100 an ounce.

With respect to ginseng in general, the following observations are generally true:

1. The whole, intact root (including the rhizome) generally commands a higher price because the buyer is better able to see what he is buying. The age of the root can be estimated by observing the number of scars on the rhizome (one for each year's growth) and the length of the rhizome (the longer it is, the older the specimen). The number of rings at the top of the root and the size of the root also are indicative of its age. In general, the older the root is, the more it is worth. Also, there is always a possibility that other forms of ginseng (powder, extract, and so on) may be "cut" with other substances that are not ginseng.

51

2. In general, a pungent odor indicates good ginseng.

Aside from the above criteria for determining the quality of ginseng, the following list explains some of the more widely used gradations of ginseng:

san-sam: This is a rare variety of Oriental wild ginseng that is near extinction. It is believed that *san-sam,* which once grew in many parts of Asia, can only be found now in certain mountainous areas of Siberia. One such root, on display in Moscow, is valued at approximately $25,000. There are many legends concerning Oriental wild ginseng. It is thought that a single dose administered sparingly causes the individual to lose consciousness, break out in severe skin eruptions, and be extremely ill for about a month. The illness gradually subsides, leaving the person healthier than he ever was previously. Any illness from which he might have been suffering vanishes entirely. This type of ginseng never finds its way out of the Orient. Many wealthy Orientals would be more than willing to spend a fortune for a genuine specimen of *san-sam,* if they could be assured of its authenticity.

kirin (Imperial Chinese ginseng): The ancient emperors of China took the very finest specimens of *san-sam* ginseng, and carefully hybridized them over many generations in order to produce the world's finest grade of cultivated ginseng. For centuries, this was the royal crop for use by the Chinese emperor, his family, and his friends. *If* the crop was plentiful enough that there was an excess, the remainder was sold to the public at enormous prices. The best specimens could command as much as six hundred times their weight in silver. It is believed that Mao Tse Tung, chairman of the Chinese Communist Party, uses *kirin* ginseng. This surprising fact was brought to light following President Nixon's visit to mainland China. The grade of ginseng used by Mao Tse Tung is probably worth about $100 an ounce.

yung sum: This is a cultivated variety of ginseng from China, although its value does not approach that of genuine *kirin* ginseng.

Korea yung sum: This is the Chinese term for cultivated Korean ginseng. In Korea, it is referred to as *insam.* This includes many different grades of ginseng. White ginseng from Korea includes *song-sam* (produced in Songto), *yong-sam* (produced in Yong-san), and *kamsan,* a peculiar type of ginseng with a crooked appearance produced in the city of Kamsan. Red ginseng produced in Korea is referred to as *hong-sam.*

far kee yung sum: This refers to the American ginseng that is imported into the Orient. It is generally considered of less value than Oriental ginseng, due to a widespread belief that the North American climate is less conducive to producing potent ginseng than the Oriental climate.

The Ginseng of Korea

The following passage appeared in *Foreign Relations of the United States* for 1886. Written by Ensign George C. Foulk of the United States Navy, it remains one of the best and most complete descriptions of the various grades of Korean ginseng in existence:

The ginseng of Corea is held by the Chinese to be the best in the world. They have used the root for many hundreds of years, as a strengthening medicine, place the most extraordinary value upon it, and seek for it in all parts of the world they visit; viewing its efficacy from their standpoint, they may therefore be well able to make this comparative estimation. Ginseng is found in China, but that there produced is considered inferior to the common marketable article in Corea. The sale of it is and has been a monopoly of the Corean government, but as might be supposed in the case of a medicine so highly necessary as it is to the Chinese, immense amounts of it have been smuggled out of Corea in all kinds of ingenious ways across the northwestern border and by junks from the west coast.

The Corean name for the root is 'Sam,' used with prefixes 'In' (man) and 'San' (mountain) respectively, to distinguish the variety cultivated by man from that found growing wild in dark mountain recesses. San-sam is extremely rare; many natives have never seen it, and it is said to be worth fully its weight in gold. This kind of ginseng is sold by the single root,

PAPERS

RELATING TO THE

FOREIGN RELATIONS

OF

THE UNITED STATES,

TRANSMITTED TO CONGRESS,

WITH THE ANNUAL MESSAGE OF THE PRESIDENT,

DECEMBER 8, 1885,

PRECEDED BY A

LIST OF PAPERS, WITH AN ANALYSIS OF THEIR CONTENTS, AND
FOLLOWED BY AN ALPHABETICAL INDEX OF SUBJECTS.

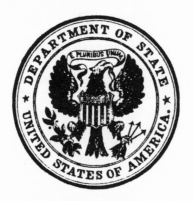

WASHINGTON:
GOVERNMENT PRINTING OFFICE.
1886.

the price of which is said to have reached in the past nearly $2,000 for an extraordinarily fine large specimen. The san-sam root is much larger than any cultivated variety, its length ranging from a foot to three and four, with a thickness at the head of from 1½ to 2½ inches. At the top of the root proper and base of the stem of the plant is a corky section of rings, the number of which shows the age of the root. The seed of san-sam, planted in the mountains under circumstances similar to those under which the mother plant grew, will produce a root somewhat like true san-sam, and in this way imitation san-sam it produced; but an effort to sell it as san-sam is regarded as a swindle, and it is said that experts readily perceive that it has been produced by the aid of man. It is believed that the virtues of san-sam do not lie in the material composition of the plant, but are due to a mysterious power attached to it by being produced wholly apart from man's influence, under the care of a beneficient spirit or god. True san-sam is supposed never even to have been seen by man while it was attaining the state in which it was found. Twenty, thirty, and forty years have been named to me as the ages of certain san-sam plants when found.

The san-sam root is carefully taken from the earth when found, carefully washed and gently scraped, then thoroughly sun-dried. In administering it, the whole root is eaten as one dose, it may be in two parts. The person then becomes unconscious (some people here say dies) and remains so three days. After this the whole body is full of ills for about a month, then rejuvenation begins, the skin becomes clear, the body healthy, and the person will henceforth live, free from sickness, suffering neither heat nor cold until he has attained the age of ninety or an hundred years.

The extreme rarity of san-sam augments the superstitious repute in which it is held; as an intelligent Corean told me, much that is said of it is only words; nevertheless, he maintained that san-sam was a wonderful medicine in its strengthening effects.

Insam, the cultivated ginseng of Corea; is produced in large quantity, and is a common marketable article. While it is most highly appreciated by the Chinese, it is also believed to be the best of medicines by the Coreans. It is nearly all produced in two distant sections of Corea, viz, at Songto (Kai-seng), about 60 miles to the north and westward of the capital, and at Yong-san, in Kyung-sang-do, the southeasternmost province of Corea. The qualities produced in these two sections are regarded as differing, and the ginseng is known as Song-sam, or Yong-sam, according as to whether it comes from Songto or Yong-sam, in Kyung-san-do, respectively. The former place I visited recently and in the company of a government official inspected several of the principle farms.

Foulk then gives us a rare description of the method by which red ginseng is made. Red ginseng refers to a specially cured form of ginseng that is made from fresh white roots. Red ginseng has the advantage of being preserved indefinitely, and it cannot be attacked by insects. On the other hand, there is a tiny pest known as the boring beetle that can attack even perfectly dried *white* roots. This pest can be detected by the presence of tiny white larvae which make little burrows throughout the roots. The red ginseng roots, however, are immune from attack by this pest.

In addition to being preserved, red ginseng roots are thought by some to be more potent than white ginseng of comparable grade.

The roots have a reddish translucent appearance, somewhat resembling hard candy in consistency. The usual method of taking red ginseng is to bite off a small piece and retain it in the mouth. Used in this manner, a small amount will go a long way. The process of making red ginseng is described by Foulk as follows:

Soon after the seeds have been gathered in October the plants and roots intact are carefully taken from the earth. The stems are readily broken off, the roots washed, placed in small baskets with large meshes, and at once taken to the steaming house. Here are flat, shallow iron boilers over fire places, over which are earthenware vessels 2 feet in diameter and as many high with close-fitting lids. In the bottoms of the earthenware vessels are five holes 2 inches in diameter. Water is boiled in the iron vessels, the steam rising and filling the upper vessels through these holes.

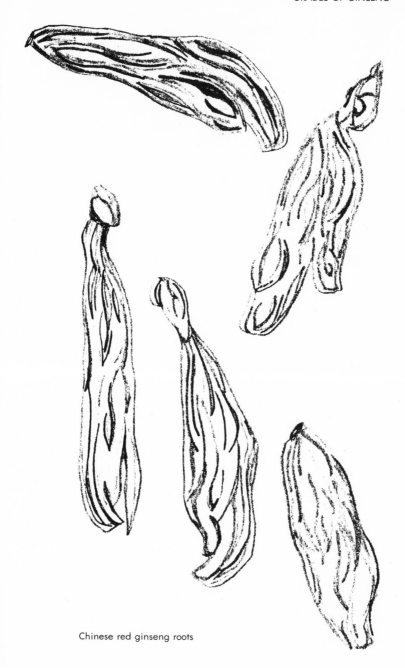

Chinese red ginseng roots

The small baskets containing the roots having been placed in the earthenware vessel and the latter tightly closed, the steaming process goes on for from one and a half to four hours, when the roots are removed and taken to the drying house. This is a long building containing racks of bamboo poles, on which in rows are placed flat drying baskets. Under the floor of the house, at intervals of 3 or 4 feet, are fire places, the smoke from which passes out of small holes in the back of the house under the floor level. In the baskets of the drying house the roots are spread and the fires kept going constantly for about ten days, when the roots are supposed to be cured. From here they are packed for the market in rectangular willow baskets closely lined with paper to exclude moisture.

During this process the roots become very toughly hard, and their color changes from carroty white to nearly cherrywood red. They break hard but crisply, exhibiting a shiny, glassy fracture, translucent, dark red. The ginseng resulting from this process is called hong-sam (red ginseng), and is the article prohibited from export from Corea in all the treaties made by Corea with the Western Powers. It is the most common ginseng seen in Corea, and by far the majority of it is produced in the Songto section.

Foulk concludes with an interesting discussion of "Pak-sam," the various methods of using ginseng in Korea, and the ginseng trade in Primorskaya.

'Pak-sam' is insam simply washed, scraped, and sun-dried after being taken from the earth. This kind is much used domestically, but not having been cured will not bear exportation. It is regarded by many as better medicine than hong-sam, and is occasionally, depending upon form and quality, higher in price consequently.

The ways of using insam are many. Most commonly, cut or broken into small pieces, it is mixed with other medicines to form pills, tablets, decoctions to be drunk, and so on. Some times the plain root is eaten dry. This is very common.

Old people make a warm decoction by boiling the simple root cut in pieces. It would seem to be regarded as a strengthening medicine for every part of the system. The shape of the root is commonly likened to that of a man, a consequence of its four distinct shape sections. By some people each of these different parts of the man is believed to be adapted to a particular complaint; thus the head to eye affections, the body to general debility, the arms and legs to stomach disorders, colds, and female disorders. This man shape of the root figures largely in the purchase of certain kinds of ginseng, especially with that of san-sam.

A rival of Korea in supplying ginseng for the Chinese market is Primorskaya, province of Siberia, in the vicinity of Vladivostok. About here great numbers of Chinese congregate in search of it. Near one place, to the northeastward of Vladivostok, Souchan, and on the Danbihe River it is cultivated quite largely by them. The various nomadic tribes in eastern Siberia seek for san-sam in the mountains, and in its sale, together with that of sable skins, find their living.

The method of cultivation given above is that explained to me at one of the ginseng farms in Songto; I have been told, however, that there are other slightly different methods followed in different places and by different farmers. Some roots are fit for market in five and a half or six years after planting, but to produce the best article, seven years' growth is necessary. The market price of red ginseng (hong-sam) is at present nearly $4 per English pound.

In addition to red ginseng, there is also a less common form of sugar-cured ginseng that is popular in some parts of the Orient. The fresh roots are first thoroughly cleaned and washed. Then they are coated with a hot sugary solution; white sugar for a light color, brown sugar for a darker color. The roots are then placed over boiling water and steamed. As they are being steamed, some of the sugar is absorbed; the remainder falls to the bottom of the pots. The sugar that falls to the bottom is recrystallized into "ginseng sugar," which actually does have the taste of ginseng. During the steaming process, the roots are coated with the hot sugary solution several times. They are later removed and placed in the sun to dry.

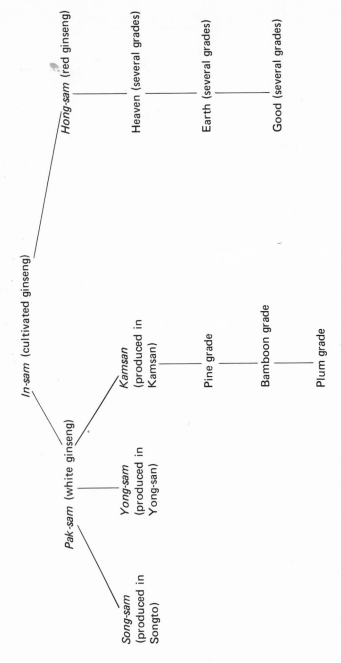

In-sam (cultivated ginseng)

Pak-sam (white ginseng)

Hong-sam (red ginseng)

Song-sam (produced in Songto)

Yong-sam (produced in Yong-san)

Kamsan (produced in Kamsan)

Pine grade

Bamboon grade

Plum grade

Heaven (several grades)

Earth (several grades)

Good (several grades)

Note: Heaven, Earth, and God grades are sometimes used to categorize *Pak-sam* (white ginseng).

Grades of Cultivated Korean Ginseng

Korean Red Ginseng

There are many grades of Korean red ginseng. The three basic grades are Heaven (first grade), Earth (second grade), and Good (third grade). Within each of the three basic grades, there are numerous sub-grades, summarized as follows:

Grade	Approximate Weight of 1 Root
Heaven 10	1.20 oz.
Heaven 20	0.75 oz.
Heaven 30	0.55 oz.
Heaven 40	0.45 oz.
Heaven 50	0.35 oz.
Earth 10	1.45 oz.
Earth 20	1.00 oz.
Earth 30	0.80 oz.
Earth 40	0.70 oz.
Good 20	1.25 oz.
Good 30	0.80 oz.

A root is placed in one of the three grades on the basis of its shape, texture, and color. It is then placed in one of the sub-grades on the basis of weight.

The Chinese include *all* of the grades mentioned above in one Chinese grade, *Korea yung sum*.

Kamsan Ginseng

Kamsan is a special grade of ginseng that comes from a city of the same name in Korea. It refers to a variety of white ginseng that is unusually crooked in appearance, unlike the normally straight appearance of ginseng roots. It is further divided into four sub-grades, determined primarily on the basis of size. The larger a root

61

is, the higher its grade. In order of decreasing value, the grades are as follows:

Kamsan, Pine Grade (largest)

Kamsan, Bamboon Grade

Kamsan, Plum Grade (smallest)

Because a straight ginseng root more closely resembles the human body than a crooked root, *Kamsan* is generally considered slightly inferior to the more straight varieties. This judgment is based entirely on the shape of the root, rather than on its medicinal properties as such.

Japanese Ginseng

Japanese ginseng *(Chosen-ninjin)* refers to the ginseng that is native Japan, *Panax schinseng* var. *japonicus.* This variety has never been held in high esteem by ginseng users; in fact, it is considered the poorest grade of ginseng available. Dr. I. J. Shephard explains the situation:

> The last and poorest quality is the Japanese ginseng, which, like the native product, is used for the adulteration of the Korean supply and other better grades.

However, Japanese ginseng is used as an aromatic tonic, and is regarded as a good medicine for heart ailments.

Perhaps one reason that Japanese ginseng is held in such low esteem is that the roots often grow horizontally rather than vertically. Thus, they rarely have the humanoid appearance so desired by ginseng users. This is partly a reflection on the fact that much of Japan is covered with poor, rocky soil which makes irregular roots inevitable.

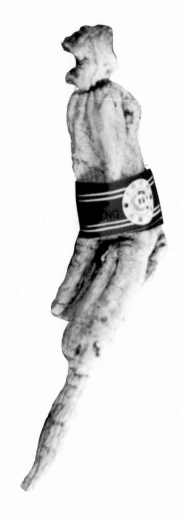

Korean Ginseng Root

Eleutherococcus senticosus

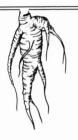

"Siberian Ginseng"

The Soviet Union has done considerable research on the medicinal plants of the Far East. This research has recently brought to light a very potent plant in the ginseng family, *Eleutherococcus senticosus*, which is also known as "Siberian ginseng."

Eleutherococcus is about ten feet tall when full grown, unlike ginseng which seldom exceeds a foot in height. As with ginseng, the root is the part of the plant that is used medicinally. It is usually administered as an extract or as a tincture.

In many ways, *Eleutherococcus* produces effects similar to those of ginseng. However, there are some notable differences. *Eleutherococcus* has been shown to increase physical capacity for work longer and somewhat more effectively than ginseng. It has also been shown to be of greater value in the treatment of radiation sickness, cancer, and certain types of diabetes, in some early and inconclusive studies. Also, it is believed that *Eleutherococcus* is somewhat more effective than ginseng in combating the adverse effects of stress.

Like ginseng, *Eleutherococcus* produces definite anabolic effects in healthy organisms. In a recent animal study, mice that were fed

Eleutherococcus remained in heat 50 percent longer than the control group. Also, they had substantially more offspring than those in the control group, a direct effect of more frequent sexual activity. Also, the mice that were born to parents that were given *Eleutherococcus* weighed more, and were less prone to infant mortality.

Similar experiments have not yet been performed on humans to determine the effects of *Eleutherococcus* on fertility, although an anabolic effect on humans is evident on the basis of blood and urine tests.

Eleutherococcus extract is widely used in the Soviet Union, and it is exported to the United States. Sources for this product are given in *The Herb Buyer's Guide.*

Botany of *Eleutherococcus*

Eleutherococcus senticosus is a member of the Araliaciae family, to which ginseng also belongs. It is sometimes called *Acanthopanax senticosus,* and occasionally *Aralia manchuria.*

It grows wild in far eastern Russia, Korea, and northern China. It is usually found in forest clearings, either singly or in small groups. It has the appearance of a large shrub, six to fifteen feet in height. The branches are covered with a wrinkled bark on which there are numerous prickly thorns. New shoots originate from buds found on the roots, or from the upper parts of pre-existing branches. The leaves are composed of three to five leaflets, each of which varies in length from three to five inches. The leaves are doubly serrate and bright green; the bottoms are smooth or partially covered with brown hairs. The stems of the leaves have a thin covering of brown fuzz, and are thorny. The flowers are borne in clusters, several at the ends of the branches. The flowers are small, with yellowish-white petals. They give rise to very dark blue berries (almost black), each of which contains about five seeds. The plant flowers in July and August; the fruit matures in October. It is deciduous and loses its leaves annually.

Eleutherococcus reproduces itself by seed, by new shoots which originate from buds found on the roots, or by layering. Layering refers to a method of reproduction in which a branch becomes partially buried in the soil while it is still attached to the plant. Roots begin to form where the branch is buried. When the roots are large enough, the new plant can be safely severed from the mother plant.

For many years, botanists were unable to germinate the seeds of *Eleutherococcus* under artificial conditions. Then, a very interesting discovery was made. In nature, after the seeds fall to the ground, they must be eaten by a bird and pass through its digestive tract before they can germinate. It was found that the hydrochloric acid in the birds' stomachs is necessary to initiate the germination process. Thus, the seeds must now be treated with dilute hydrochloric acid in order for them to germinate under artificial conditions. Only a brief exposure to the acid is necessary. This seems to serve the purpose of softening the very hard seed coat, so that water can penetrate into the seed and begin the germination process.

Natural Habitats of Asiatic Ginseng and *Eleutherococcus*

Eleutherococcus senticosus was first discovered in the wild state in the Primorye territory of Siberia. It is presently under cultivation in this area, and wild specimens can still be found.

Wild *Panax schinseng* is very nearly an extinct article of the Asian continent. It is not fully known exactly where the original native habitat of this plant was, because it has been gathered in the wild for many centuries.

On the basis of the somewhat fragmentary material that has been handed down from the past, the most likely places where ginseng once grew wild would be the following: in the mountains of Nepal (near India's northern border), and in the region extending from the eastern extremity of the Plateau of Tibet, through Manchuria and the southeastern end of Siberia.

Although the above regional boundaries are estimated on the basis of information handed down from the past, it is known with certainty that wild ginseng is found today only in the north eastern part of China, northern Korea, and in the Sikhote-Alin Mountains of

67

Siberia. In these areas, it is extremely rare, and bordering on extinction.

Wild ginseng from the Sikhote-Alin Mountains is considered by many to be the finest grade in the world. Also, it is the most expensive grade.

Eleutherococcus a Menace?

When the Russian government first began to study *Eleutherococcus senticosus*, they did so because certain tribes in Siberia had used the plant medicinally for centuries. Russian researchers wanted to know why the plant was held in such high esteem. There was, however, one group that did not use *Eleutherococcus*. In fact, this group considered the plant a thorny menace. It was the "Gold"—the people of the Manchurian branch of the Tungus-Manchurian tribe—who regarded *Eleutherococcus* as an annoying menace while hunting for ginseng!

Eleutherococcus senticosus is a very thorny plant that becomes dry and brittle during the winter. At this time, it is hard to spot; but the thorns are very treacherous to anyone that inadvertently brushes against the plant. They have a tendency to break off when they are in this brittle state, and to remain in the skin like nasty splinters.

Although the plant grows in many parts of the Far East, it is particularly abundant in the Sikhote-Alin Mountains where wild Asiatic ginseng is occasionally found also. In wandering through the dense forests of these mountains, it was only too easy to run into *Eleutherococcus*, which at that time had no real market value. The peasants of the region who used it merely went out and gathered some from time to time. It was possible to gather *Eleutherococcus* without having to venture into the high mountainous areas.

In the ginseng plantations of far eastern Russia, *Eleutherococcus* was regarded as the most annoying of all the "weeds" that plagued these plantations.

Now that a considerable market for *Eleutherococcus* has arisen, it is doubtful that this plant is regarded as a "weed" at all any more.

Nevertheless, the price of wild *Eleutherococcus* has never even approached the price of wild Asiatic ginseng, because *Eleutherococcus* is far more abundant than wild Asiatic ginseng.

Although *Eleutherococcus senticosus* may be sold in the United States for beverage purposes, it is against the law to make any medicinal claims for it in this country at the present time. After further research has been conducted, the Food and Drug Administration may approve its use for specific medical purposes.

Other countries, however, have already approved *Eleutherococcus* for use in a large variety of ailments. Here is the prescribing information as it appears in other countries:

FLUID EXTRACT OF ELEUTHEROCOCCUS
(Extractum Eleutherococci Fluidum)

Extractum Eleutherococci Fluidum is an extract of the rhizomes of thorny *Eleutherococcus (Eleutherococcus senticosus)*.

It is a nontransparent liquid of dark brown color with specific slightly burning taste and a characteristic odor.

The preparation is of low toxicity, improves the general physical condition, and exerts a tonic effect. It increases physical and mental work capacity as well as resistivity of the organism to different untoward influences and diseases.

Extractum Eleutherococci Fluidum reduces hyperglycemia, normalizes the blood pressure, improves appetite and sleep.

Indications:

Overstrain of organism

Convalescence after a serious illness or operation

Prolonged diseases accompanied by exhaustion of organism

Functional disorder of nervous system, weakness, various kinds of neuroses, hypertonia, and hypotonia

Initial stages of atherosclerosis

Mild to moderate cases of diabetes

69

Dosages:

> 20 to 40 drops or three times daily for a period of 30 days. May be repeated after 10-15 days, if necessary.

Contraindications:

> Hypertonic crisis, myocardial infarcation.

Eleutherococcus and the Treatment of Mental Illness

Preparations of *Eleutherococcus senticosus* seem to be especially valuable in the treatment of adverse mental states that originate from both phychological and physical causes.

In the treatment of patients who have suffered brain concussions, *Eleutherococcus* often lessens the normal recovery time. It has also been shown to be highly useful in the treatment of asthenic states, which are abnormal states of mind in which weakness and debility predominate, and are fairly noticeable. There are many ways in which asthenia manifests itself, including excessive fatigue, faintness, dizziness, and muscular pain. Asthenia can only be diagnosed by a physician. It is not actually a disease in itself, but a pathological state that can accompany a number of different illness. Also, it can be produced by any of several different causes. Asthenia sometimes accompanies schizophrenia. More commonly, it might follow a severe case of influenza.

Perhaps a clue to the way in which *Eleutherococcus* alleviates asthenic states can be found in the fact that an insufficiency of the adrenal cortex can cause this condition. If the adrenal cortex is overworked, or if it is unable to function properly for any reason, asthenia will result. It is known that ginseng and *Eleutherococcus* have a strenghtening effect on the adrenal cortex. Thus, it is not surprising that ginseng and *Eleutherococcus* would also help to relieve asthenia.

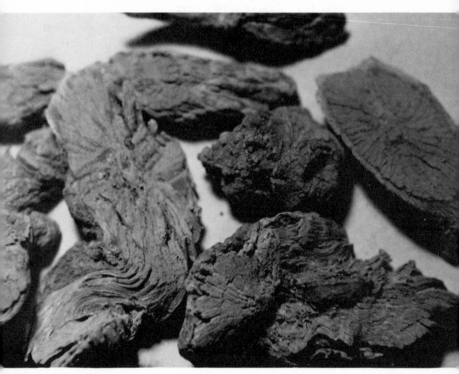

erococcus Root Slices

The Use of Asiatic Ginseng

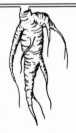

Ginseng and the *Yang* Element

According to Chinese philosophy, a healthy body contains a balance of two universal elements—the *yin* and the *yang*. There is no way to define these two terms precisely, because there are no words in the English language that mean *yin* or *yang* exactly. They are two opposite forces; *yin* is characterized by femininity, coldness, inward movement; *yang* is characterized by masculinity, warmth, outward movement. *Yin* corresponds to the heavens; yang corresponds to the Earth.

In order to fully understand the Chinese concept of ginseng, one must first understand the concept of *yin* and *yang*. This is because ginseng is considered a strongly *yang* medicine. It is considered to be of masculine gender; hence the word ginseng means "man-image," literally. Ginseng is also regarded as a strongly "heating" medicine. All *yang* medicines are considered "heating;" all *yin* medicines are "cooling."

In accordance with the philosophy of *yin* and *yang,* disease is caused either by an overabundance of the *yin* element, or by the overabundance of the *yang* element. In the healthy body, the two elements are in perfect balance.

Some Chinese physicians feel that Americans, in general, possess too much of the *yang* element, and should therefore use moderation in the use of ginseng (which is a *yang* medicine).*

*If a person has too much *yang*, he is typically prone to swellings and ulcers, vascular disorders (including heart disease), muscular and skeletal problems, and gastrointestinal disorders. Nevertheless, modern studies have shown that ginseng (a *yang* medicine) is useful in all of these conditions.

In the context of what has just been explained, the following passage can be much better understood. It was written over a century ago by an early French explorer in China. Keep in mind that "heating" and "hot" refer to the concept of *yin* and *yang*.

> Jin-seng is perhaps the most considerable article of Man-tchourian commerce. Throughout China there is no chemist's shop unprovided with more or less of it.
>
> The root of jin-seng is straight, spindle-shaped, and very knotty; seldom so large as one's little finger, and in length from two to three inches. When it has undergone its fitting preparation, its colour is a transparent white, with sometimes a slight red or yellow tinge. Its appearance, then, is that of a branch of stalactite.
>
> The Chinese report marvels of the jin-seng, and no doubt it is, for Chinese organization, a tonic of very great effect for old and weak persons; but its nature is too heating, the Chinese physicians admit, for the European temperament; already, in their opinion, too hot.

Ginseng and Endurance

Many people take ginseng hoping to find themselves more alert if they are tired or fatigued at the end of a hard day. They expect it to act somewhat like coffee, temporarily relieving the tired feeling and producing wakefulness. It is natural to expect this. In our modern culture, fatigue is often treated with stimulants such as caffeine (in tea and coffee), or with prescription drugs such as the amphetamines or methylphenidate.

74

Some people do, in fact, experience wakefulness and increased alertness after taking ginseng, especially in the larger dosages. However, this should not be expected. Rather than acting quickly and wearing off in a few hours, ginseng acts in a manner that may not be noticeable at first. Rather than referring to ginseng as a stimulant, it would be more accurate to say that ginseng increases *endurance*, and tends to delay or prevent exhaustion. Users of ginseng, after they have taken it regularly, often notice that they are less tired at the end of a hard week. They feel that they have more energy "left over." Many people who have busy, hectic schedules say that they are able to hold out better, and often feel less tension under pressure.

On the basis of all that is known about ginseng, it can be said that ginseng is more likely to increase stamina and endurance, rather than producing prompt, immediate stimulation.

Traditional Chinese Ginseng Preparations

Perhaps the finest work available in the English language that deals with the subject of Chinese herbs is the *Chinese Materia Medica* by Dr. F. Porter Smith. The book was written by Dr. Smith in Shanghai in 1911. A recent revision of the work by Rev. G. A. Stuart, M.D. was published in Taiwan in 1969. It is a very thorough book, and I highly recommend it.

The following is a summary of some of the medicinal preparations containing ginseng whose use in China was observed by Dr. Smith.

Date and Ginseng Pills (Tsao shen wan): a tonic medicinal preparation used for ailments of the lungs and respiratory tract. (It is traditional among the Chinese to chew most medicines that are in pill form. For this reason, they are made palatable by the addition of rice flour, honey, and other nutrient substances.)

Extract of Ginseng and Aristolochia (Shen shu kao): a tonic preparation made from four ounces of ginseng to one catty of *Aristolochia recurvilabra*. The latter ingredient is the only herb actually used as a "ginseng substitute" by the Chinese in certain preparations because it is thought to have similar properties (though somewhat weaker). *Aristolochia* is considered especially valuable in gastrointestinal disturbances, dysentry, and snake bite. It is also regarded as a fine general tonic.

Purple Clavaria Pills (Tzu chih wan): another tonic preparation, unique because this formula contains virtually every Chinese herb used as a tonic in Chinese medicine. The pills are made from purple clavaria, *Dioscorea quinqueloba, Aconitum fischeri, Thuja orientalis, Polygala reinii, Pachyma cocos, Citrus fusca, Rehmannia glutinosa, Ophiopogon spicatus, Schizandra chinensis, Pinellia tuberifera, Aconitum variegatum, Paeonia moutan,* ginseng, *Polygala sibirica,* fruits of *Polygonum hydropiper, Alisma plantago,* melon seed kernels, and honey. The principle ingredient, purple clavaria, is the very famous *Ling-chih* mushroom. According to legend, the mushroom could turn earthly vapors into a heavenly atmosphere, which always surrounded the plant.

Seven Fairies Powder (Ch'i hsien tan): a medicinal powder for external application to smallpox eruptions, or as a prophylactic against the disease. It was compounded in the following manner:

> *Astragalus hoantschy,* two ounces ginseng, one ounce licorice, one-half once *Paris polyphylla,* one ounce plum flowers, one and a half ounces *Monochasma savatieri,* one ounce one piece of human skull bone

Tincture of Panax schinseng (Jen shen chiu): a fermented mixture of ginseng and rice, not unlike sake in appearance. It was used for any kind of physical debility.

Tonic Decoction (Ssu chun tzu t'ang): a tonic medicine prepared from ginseng, *Atractylis ovata, Pachyma cocos,* dried licorice root, ginger, and dates.

Resolvent Decoction (Chih chung t'ang): a medicine employed for diseases of the internal organs; especially the heart, lungs, and spleen. It contains ginseng, *Atractylis ovata,* ginger, and licorice root.

Sixteen Herb Tea (Mu tea): a traditional tonic blend of ginseng, Ligusticum, Paeonia root, cypress, orange peel, ginger, *Rehmannia,* cinnamon, cloves, peach kernels, *Coptis,* licorice, *Cnicus, Atractylis,* moutan, and hoelen.

Ginseng Leaves (Shen lu): an emetic and expectorant. For maximum effect, the leaves should be administered in the fresh, undried state. The leaves of ginseng act very different from the root, and possess no true tonic properties.

A Method of Administration

Louise Crane, writing in *Asia and the Americas,* describes a popular Chinese method of administering ginseng to a person suffering from acute illness.

First, it is necessary to wait until the patient no longer has any fever. In order to bring the patient's temperature down to normal, there are a number of Chinese herbs that are used specifically for this purpose. Then, ginseng is incorporated into a thorough treatment regimen which includes prolonged administration of dark meat, opium, tea, and of course, ginseng.

From a medical viewpoint, the treatment bears some resemblance to methods that are used today by modern physicians. For instance, a severely debilitated patient would be encouraged, in most cases, to eat plenty of protein. Dark meat is not only a good source of protein; but it is also rich in iron, a mineral essential to normal blood formation.

Tea contains caffeine, which is an overall safe and effective stimulant if used properly. Many people rely on the caffeine in coffee or tea to wake up in the morning, or to relieve temporary drowsiness. One of its most important effects is to increase the oxygen supply to the brain, which produces increased alertness.

Opium is, of course, a dangerous drug that can only be administered by a duly licensed physician. Although opium is used infrequently by modern physicians, few physicians would want to practice medicine without using some *opiates* in their practice (such as codeine, morphine, and meperidine). Used with discrete moderation, they are immensely valuable in illnesses characterized by moderate to severe pain.

In treating acute illnesses, modern doctors use substances that are basically equivalent to dark meat, opium, and tea. They do not, of course, use ginseng, or the substances contained in ginseng. If ginseng were added to the usual treatment regimen, perhaps it would favorably improve the course of many illnesses; or perhaps it would help to speed the recovery process in some cases.

A Comparison of the Dried Root vs. the Fresh Root

For most people, it is naturally very difficult to obtain fresh, undried ginseng roots. One way is to buy the live plants from mail order nurseries. Then it would be necessary to use the roots right away, or to freeze them for later use. Fresh ginseng roots are as perishable as most ordinary fresh produce items. The transportation of fresh roots over large distances—to the Orient for instance—would be extremely costly. It would entail the use of refrigerated airplanes, which would increase the cost of an already expensive article to astronomical levels.

However, there is a definite need to conduct much more research into the similarities and differences between fresh and dried ginseng roots. It is a known fact that fresh ginseng roots contain a volatile oil which is sometimes referred to as panasen. Panasen is believed to exert a direct stimulant action on the brain, somewhat like caffeine. When the roots are dried out, a large amount of the panasen initially present evaporates.

A similar situation exists in the case of a plant native to Ethiopia and parts of northern Africa. The plant I am referring to is *Catha edulis,* commonly known as khat. It is sold in the market places of Ethiopia and neighboring areas; it is very popular as a stimulant and for the alleviation of fatigue. For many years, researchers were unable to isolate the principal active ingredient in khat. In all of the investigations, however, the researchers made the mistake of studying only the dried leaves of *Catha edulis.* Recently, a French research team found that the principal active ingredient is a very volatile substance that is present only in the fresh leaves; it is entirely lost when the leaves are dried out.

The purpose of the example I have just given is simply to demonstrate the importance of studying all medicinal plants in both the fresh and dried states. Otherwise, there is no real way of knowing what important substances might be lost in the drying process.

We have reason to suspect that fresh ginseng may be somewhat more potent than the dried form. Fresh ginseng has a higher content of panasen. Also, it seems to have stronger stomachic properties if taken fresh. The fresh root also tastes considerably more pungent, somewhat like a radish. It has a slight local anaesthetic effect that leaves the mouth feeling just slightly numb a moment after it is chewed. It also leaves a faint sweet aftertaste.

The Use of Ginseng In the Near East

According to some very early accounts, wild ginseng once grew in the Himalaya Mountains in Nepal (a small nation on India's northern border). If it grows there today, it has managed to elude discovery in recent times.

Nevertheless, it has been used to some extent in India and other countries of the Middle East. An anonymous author, writing in 1895, describes the use of ginseng in that region of the world:

> In India, Persia, and Afghanistan, ginseng is known as *chob-chini,* the 'Chinese wood.' In these countries it is prepared either as a powder, which is compounded of ginseng, with gum-mastic and sugar candy, equal parts of each, about a drachm being taken once a day, early in the morning, or as a decoction, in the preparation of which an ounce of fine parings is boiled for a quarter of an hour in a pint of water. There are two ways in which the tonic is taken. The first is a truly Oriental luxurious method, affected by wealthy people, and especially by Afghan princes. The patient retires to a garden where his senses are soothed by listening to music, the song of birds, and the bubbling of a flowing stream, and enjoying the balmy breeze. He avoids everything likely to trouble and annoy him, and will not even open a letter lest it should contain bad news; and the doctor forbids anyone to contradict him. Some grandees of central Asia go through a course of forty days of this pleasant regimen every second year. The other and more commonplace method of taking ginseng requires no other precautions than the avoidance of acids, salt, and pepper, and choosing summertime, as cold is supposed to cause rheumatism.

Ginseng is also mentioned in the sacred *Atherva Veda* of ancient India:

> (Ginseng) helps bring forth seed that is poured into the female, that forsooth is the way to bring forth a son—the strength of the bull ginseng bestows on him. This herb will make you so full of lusty strength that you will, when excited, exhale heat as a thing on fire.

The Use of North American Ginseng

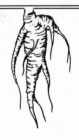

Ginseng and the Cherokees

There is an amazing similarity between the role of ginseng in the Cherokee culture, and the role of ginseng among the Asiatic ginseng prospectors.

To the Cherokee medicine men, ginseng was "Little Man," a direct reference to the sometimes humanoid appearance of the root.

Just as the Oriental prospectors believe that ginseng can hide from an unworthy pursuer and make itself invisible, such also is the belief of the Cherokee medicine men. They believe that ginseng has a mind of its own, and has the power to hide from evil men.

In gathering ginseng, a Cherokee will deliberately bypass the first three roots he encounters, and take the fourth one he finds. This is because the number four has a special magical significance for the Cherokees. Taking the fourth plant insures its efficacy as a medicine.

Before removing the ginseng plant, the finder first apologizes to the plant for what he is about to do, and a bead is placed in the hole from which the root is removed as atonement to the Plant Spirit. Amazingly, a very similar procedure is followed by the Asian ginseng hunters. They, too, say prayers of atonement for having to unearth the ginseng. Sometimes, a small altar is erected of branches and stones at the place where the root has been discovered.

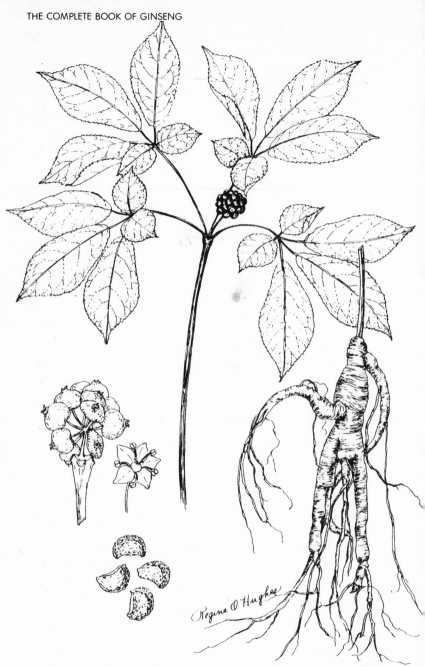

Branch, root, flower, berries, and seeds of American ginseng.

To the Cherokees, ginseng is considered an especially valuable medicine for headaches. For this purpose, the medicine man performs a small ritual which includes singing, rubbing the patient's forehead with the palm of his hand, and applying a concoction of ginseng to the areas where pain is felt.

For a condition whose description is suggestive of apoplexy, a decoction of ginseng and wild tobacco *(Nicotiana glauca)* is used. It is considered a very powerful medicine which can save the patient's life if administered in time.

Ginseng In the Chippewa Culture

The Chippewa Indians believed that ginseng, properly administered, could prolong the life of a dying person. In this they resembled the Chinese, who believed that the administration of ginseng to a dying person could prolong his life long enough for him to settle his estate and attend to his will.

It is traditional among the Chippewas to sing a song called *The White Sun-Lady* in the presence of the person who is dying, and then to blow through a reed into a decoction of ginseng. The dying person is then instructed to drink the decoction.

The person performing the ceremony addresses the soul of the dying person directly, asking it to stay rather than depart.

Use of Ginseng by the Creeks

The Creek Indians of southern Alabama and northern Florida valued ginseng very highly, and used it both as a medicine and as a magical charm.

They called it *hilis hatki,* meaning "white Medicine." It was used to treat fevers and shortness of breath, and was also included in many different medicinal preparations.

It was used in magic primarily to ward off evil spirits. The Creeks believed that a common cause of illness was contact with an evil spirit. As a preventative to this, an Indian passing by a graveyard was admonished to carry some ginseng with him, bite off a piece, and chew it. He would then spit out the ginseng first to one side, then to the other, until he had spit four times in both directions.

If an Indian was shot and seriously injured, ginseng was immediately administered in order to sustain his life long enough for him to receive proper medical treatment. The medicine man, placing bits of sliced ginseng in a cup of water, would implore Yahola, the god of physical and mental strength, to restore the patient.

John R. Swanton gives the following account of some other Creek uses of ginseng:

> When a person was sick with fever and could not sweat new ginseng was boiled with ginger, then both were mixed with alcohol and a little given to the patient, when sweat would break out all over him. It was also used, according to both Caley Proctor and Jackson Lewis, to stop the flow of blood from a cut. The latter by its means cured a woman who had been shot in the head. Before applying the medicine in such cases the wound was cleaned out by the use of the long wing feather of a buzzard.

Ginseng and the Mide Indians

Ginseng was used by the Mide Indians of the northwestern United States in a way that was strangely similar to the use of *Panax schinseng* in the Orient.

Medicinally, it was considered an excellent remedy for every kind of stomach ailment.

Another use involved the administration of those parts of the root that resembled the afflicted part of the patient's body (c.f. Doctrine of Signatures). In other words, the "arm" of the root would be used to treat arm afflictions, and so on. In Mide tradition, ginseng (called *Shte-na-bi-o-dzhi-bik*) means "man-root." It was one of the "great medicines," a gift from the Mide Spirit. One legend describes its use in bringing a dead boy back to life. There is no doubt that it was a medicine highly esteemed by the Mide medicine men.

A Pawnee Love Charm

The Pawnee Indians of northern Oklahoma used ginseng in combination with several other herbs to produce a love charm. The following account appeared in the *Thirty-Third Annual Report of the American Bureau of Ethnology:*

> A Pawnee gave the information that ginseng roots in composition with certain other substances were used as a love charm. From various individuals the information was gathered bit by bit severally and adduced, showing that the four species of plants used in compounding the love charm were *Aquilegia canadensis, Lobelia cardinalis, Cogswellia daucifolia,* and *Panax quinquefolium,* or possibly a species of *Ligusticum.* Specimens of the latter were not in hand, but informants spoke of it as *Angelica.* They had become acquainted with *Angelica* of the pharmacists and probably mistook it for their own native *Ligusticum.* It is possible that various combinations of four plants might have been used, but it appears certain that *Aquilegia canadensis* and *Cogswellia daucifolia* were considered most potent. The parts used were the seeds of *Aquilegia* and *Cogswellia,* dried roots of *Panax,* and dried roots and flowers of *Lobelia cardinalis.* With these vegetal products was mingled red-earth paint. The possession of these medicines was supposed to invest the possessor with a property of attractiveness to all persons, in spite of any natural antipathy which might otherwise exist. When to these were added hairs obtained by stealth through the friendly offices of an amiably disposed third person from the head of the woman who was desired, she was unable to resist the attraction and soon yielded to the one who possessed the charm.

Ginseng and the Sioux Indians

The Sioux Indians never used ginseng very extensively; at any rate, they never considered it a panacea. Nevertheless, they were very much involved in the gathering and preparation of the roots for export. They worked in collaboration with the International Ginseng

Company of New York, which purchased their ginseng and exported it.

In the Orient, Sioux ginseng brought unusually large prices and was generally valued more than ordinary gathered North American roots. The Sioux had a special method of curing the roots that is still only partially known to the outside world.

In cleaning the roots, the Indians placed them in barrels of water and thoroughly agitated them by rotating rods that were diagonally positioned in the barrels. According to the Sioux, this technique cleaned the roots even more thoroughly than if each root were to be brushed by hand. At the same time, there was no danger of damaging even the most delicate parts of the roots.

Sioux ginseng was not so much valued because of its cleanliness, but because of its rich, translucent color. This technique, in which translucence is imparted to the roots, remains unknown to the outside world.

Bright With Silver

At the turn of the century, four brothers embarked on a daring adventure designed to make profitable their parents' remote Wisconsin farm. The plan was to raise the beautiful silver fox, which they were convinced was the world's most beautiful fur-bearing animal. Frustrated by their repeated failure to trap a silver fox, they decided to breed the animal instead from selected stock. To begin such an enterprise was expensive, however, and the Fromm brothers turned to ginseng cultivation in hopes that it would bring in enough money to support their work with the foxes.

Although ginseng growing was, and still is, a sideline to raising foxes, few have had more success in that area than the Fromm brothers. At the present time, they are the largest North American producers of ginseng for export to the Orient.

An excellent account of the Fromm brothers' venture—from a small beginning to a major enterprise—is told in *Bright With Silver* by Kathrine Pinkerton. It should be read by anyone who is seriously interested in the history of ginseng cultivation in America.

Ginseng and the Edgar Cayce Formulas

Edgar Cayce, perhaps the most famous psychic medium of modern times, became world-famous for his uncanny ability to enter into a trance for the benefit of a sick person, render a diagnosis, and then prescribe the treatment.

Many of the ingredients in these remedies were unknown to Cayce and to the rest of the medical profession as well. Often, the ingredients were difficult to locate, and sometimes they would turn up in remote parts of the world. In spite of their often unusual nature, they always seemed to produce a cure. In fact, Cayce always said that if any of his treatments ever caused harm to anyone, he would permanently discontinue his work.

No one really knows just what caused the trances. Cayce himself never knew. Those who have studied the life of Edgar Cayce believe that he was somehow attuned to a "world mind"—a vast repository of medical knowledge. Some people would call this the mind of God—the Divine Physician—acting through Edgar Cayce.

At any rate, the evidence makes it very improbable that Cayce was a charlatan. While in a trance, he could speak fluidly on the same level with many of the finest medical specialists of his time. He received countless referrals from noted specialists who believed in his work.

One of the ingredients often included in the Edgar Cayce remedies was wild North American ginseng. It is interesting that he never mentioned the cultivated root, but always specified wild ginseng. In one of the Edgar Cayce readings, he referred to it as:

> · according to the Ancients, the basis of the stimulation of life in its very essence in the body of man.

According to other readings, it is said to possess definite powers of rejuvenation.

Available Edgar Cayce preparations that contain wild ginseng include *Formula 636 Tonic* (designed to improve the functioning of the glands in general and to restore color to graying hair), *Formula 208 Tonic* (for intestinal ailments), and *Passion Flower Fusion* (a mild, non habit-forming sedative).

87

A source for all of the Edgar Cayce remedies is given in *The Herb Buyer's Guide.*

Ginseng In Smoke

During the Second World War, a new idea in the manufacture of cigarettes was introduced. A company by the name of the R. L. Swain Tobacco Company introduced *Pinehurst,* a cigarette using ginseng extract as the hygroscopic agent. (Hygroscopic agents are found in practically all cigarettes. They keep the tobacco slightly moist so that it clings together.)

Due to our present stringent laws regulating the claims a manufacturer can make when it relates to a person's health, the following statement, which appeared on *Pinehurst,* might seem somewhat unrestrained. The statement, though interesting, has never been conclusively proven in laboratory and clinical experiments:

> Gin-Seng extract used exclusively by this company as a hygroscopic agent may also provide a mollifying feature which may relieve dry throat, cigarette cough, and other irritations due to smoking, and may be far more pleasant and safe for those with ordinary colds and respiratory difficulties such as hay fever, asthma, etc. Also, nicotine in smoke may be less than in many of the other popular brands as indicated by scientific test.

Illustration on next page
from *American Medicinal Plants*
by Charles F. Millspaugh.

1 and 2.   Whole plant, Pittsburgh, Pa., June 28, 1885.
      3.   Section of flower.
      4.   Part of calyx, a petal and stamen.
5 and 6.   Fruit.
      7.   Section of rhizome.

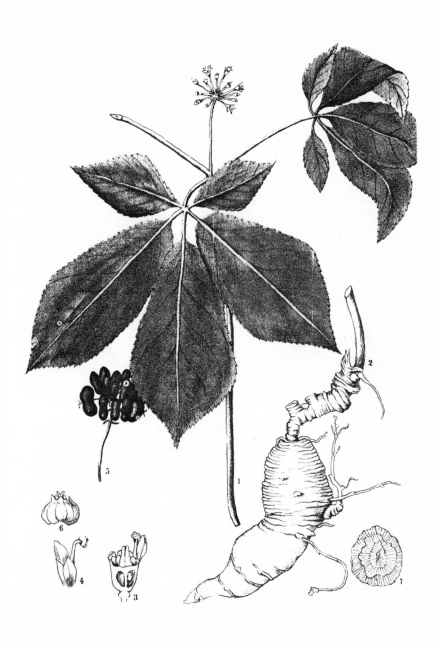

Early Research

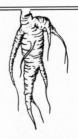

Early Research on Ginseng

In the early 1900s, two unusual research studies were performed on ginseng, both by Russian investigators working independently.

The first of these studies was performed by M. Y. Galvialo, working under the direction of Dr. A. Y. Danilevsky at the Imperial Military-Medical Academy of Russia. In describing the nature of his findings, Galvialo said that it:

> appears that the root contains a certain vegetable substance which in its chemical nature has a curious affinity with animal sperm and the active alkaloid of cola-nuts. . . . The presence of the vegetable sperm partly explains its strange effectiveness in heightening the general tone of the organism and regenerating physical vigor. . . .

It has since been learned that the active alkaloid of cola nuts is caffeine. So in effect he is saying that the substance has a "chemical affinity" with animal sperm and caffeine. Just what is meant by "affinity" in this context is not clear. Perhaps he means that a chemical reaction takes place. At any rate, Galvialo's findings remain somewhat of a mystery; it would be worthwhile for a modern investigator to study his findings and attempt to interpret them in terms of present-day knowledge.

The second study was conducted by Alexander Gurwitch in the 1920s. According to Gurwitch, ginseng emits invisible energy waves which he termed "mitogenetic radiation." He stated that ginseng continues to emit this radiation after it has been uprooted, and that this radiation has a definite hormonal effect that is beneficial to the body.

These studies also remain somewhat questionable, but not altogether impossible. Some recent studies conducted on various plants have demonstrated the possible existence of invisible radiation, such as that found in plant and animal "auras."

After these two early studies mentioned above, no further studies were conducted for many years. Just before the start of the Second World War, the Russians began some very extensive research on ginseng. However, before these studies really "got off the ground," their work was interrupted by the war. It was not resumed until the early part of the Korean War when the Russians reportedly seized the entire Korean supply of ginseng, valued at approximately $120,000,000. Needless to say, this was sufficient to provide research material for many more studies.

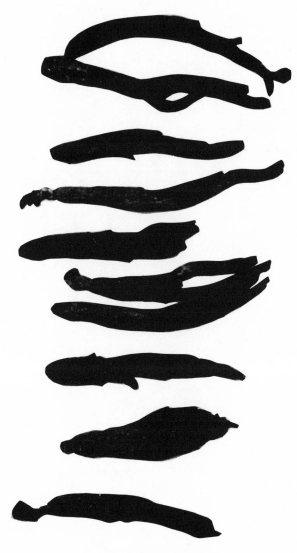

Chinese Red Ginseng Roots

Modern Research Findings

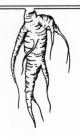

Recent Study

Certainly much additional research is needed; but on the basis of recent experiments, it would appear that ginseng and *Eleutherococcus* act in the following manner:

When the body is subjected to everyday stress, the adrenal cortex must work very hard in order to manufacture hormones so that the body can cope with the stress. When ginseng or *Eleutherococcus* are given, they seem to do the work of these hormones, so that the body does not really have to manufacture them in such large amounts. In short, the constituents of ginseng and *Eleutherococcus* seem to take the place of the hormones of the adrenal cortex. Consequently, the adrenal cortex does not become overworked.

In a similar way, the same principle is responsible for the action of antibiotics. When there is an infection somewhere in the body, the body produces antibodies and white blood cells in order to fight the infection. However, when an antibiotic is administered, the antibiotic takes the place of the antibodies and white blood cells in fighting the infection. Since the body does not have to work as hard in order to fight the infection, the individual normally gets well much faster.

In addition to the clinical evidence which seems to indicate that ginseng and *Eleutherococcus* take the place of the adrenal cortical hormones, there is also a great deal of striking evidence for this theory from a chemical standpoint. The chemical constituents have a remarkably similar appearance to the steroid hormones, which include the sex hormones, cortisone, and DCA.

The adrenal gland in man is composed, actually, of two distinct glands, each of which has its own special function. It is made up of the adrenal cortex, which is the outer shell of the adrenal gland, and the adrenal medulla, which is the inner part of the adrenal gland surrounded by the adrenal cortex. It is the adrenal cortex that we will be concerned with here because of its relation to the action of ginseng and *Eleutherococcus*.

The adrenal cortex is a vital organ without which there could be no life. It manufactures essentially three different types of hormones: (1) those that regulate sugar metabolism; (2) those that regulate the mineral content of the body tissues; and (3) sex hormones, which play a rather minor role in comparison to the sex hormones manufactured elsewhere in the body.

When a person is subjected to stress, the body reacts to this stress in the following manner: First, the pituitary gland (which seems to regulate all the other glands in the body) produces a hormone called ACTH. Then, ACTH stimulates the adrenal cortex to produce DCA and cortisone. Cortisone causes a prompt increase in the blood sugar level, so that the body (by burning sugar faster) will have sufficient energy to cope with the stressful situation. DCA, in order to make certain that the body's vital mineral balance is not disturbed while the metabolism is accelerated, serves to regulate this balance.

This "adaptive reaction" to stress is both normal and useful, because it enables the body to function at top efficiency during the stressful situation.

However, this adaptive reaction was not designed to work well under conditions of frequent or prolonged stress. When the individual is subjected to stress too frequently or for too long, a number of diverse symptoms may begin to manifest themselves. These include high blood pressure, heart disease, ulcers, anxiety, neurosis, chronic fatigue, and exhaustion. Unfortunately, modern living is notorious for exposing people to far more stress than they were built to endure. Consequently, these diseases are seen far too often.

In addition to the symptoms of too much stress described above, there are also certain signs that can be detected only in the laboratory. Four of these signs are: (1) an increase in the number of eosinophils in the outer blood vessels; (2) an increase in the weight of the adrenal glands (which is a sign that they are working very hard); (3) a decrease in the ascorbic acid content of the adrenals (because the adrenals use up their supply of ascorbic acid); and (4) a decrease in the amount of cholesterol in the adrenals.

When laboratory experiments are done with ginseng and *Eleutherococcus,* stress can be directly measured in any or all of the above ways. Of course, the tests are somewhat better suited to laboratory animals, because they can be exposed to stress, and then sacrificed in order to examine the adrenal glands more carefully. In humans, blood and urine samples are studied.

Modern research studies, many of which have been performed by the noted Dr. I. I. Brekhman, have indicated that ginseng and *Eleutherococcus* tend to prevent the normal manifestations of stress, *while enhancing the subject's ability to cope with the stressful situation.* In animal studies, mice exposed to stress show no significant increase in the number of eosinophils in the outer blood vessels, or in the weight of the adrenals. Nor do they show any significant decrease in the ascorbic acid or cholesterol content of the adrenals. Yet they consistently manage to out-perform the animals that did not receive ginseng or *Eleutherococcus.*

In one experiment, chickens were exposed to extreme cold, which normally tends to decrease their egg-laying capacity. For a period of two months, the hens were regularly exposed to the cold. One group was given a daily dose of *Eleutherococcus* extract, and the other group was not. The hens that were given *Eleutherococcus* continued to lay eggs as though they had not been exposed to cold at all. For the two month period, the hens that received *Eleutherococcus* actually laid over twice as many eggs as the control group.

In another experiment, mice were made to run on an inclined moving ramp. The mice were initially divided into two groups. One group was given *Eleutherococcus* extract for twelve days prior to the experiment; the other was not. It was found that the mice that were given prior treatment with *Eleutherococcus* were able to run on the ramp for an average of about thirty minutes before exhaustion occured. The mice that did not receive *Eleutherococcus*, however, could only stay on the ramp for about twenty minutes before becoming exhausted. In other words, the treated group was able to endure the situation 50% longer than the untreated group.

Other studies in which animals were given ginseng extract have demonstrated that the treated animals are also able to outswim, and even *outsurvive* the untreated animals. For example, laboratory rats that were not treated with ginseng lived an average of about 659 days, whereas those that were given ginseng lived an average of about 768 days. Similar tests have not yet been performed on humans, but the equivalent of this difference in humans would amount to an extension of the average lifespan by about ten years.

Constituents of Ginseng

The root of ginseng contains a resin, sugar, starch, mucilage, a saponin, a volatile oil (which might contain an unidentified central nervous system stimulant), and several steroid compounds such as panaxatriol. The activity of ginseng is primarily due to its steroid constituents.

A steroid is a chemical compound with the same basic structure as the sex hormones and the adrenal cortical hormones, of which estrogen, testosterone, cortisone, and DCA are prime examples.

Testosterone, the male sex hormone, is found in different proportions in the male and female body; and acts as the body's natural anabolic. By definition, an anabolic is a substance that builds up the general health of the body by regulating the burning of energy. The opposite of an anabolic is a catabolic which temporarily gives a person more energy, but does so by tearing down body energy reserves. Essentially, the difference between an anabolic and a catabolic (of which the drug amphetamine is a good example) is that *an anabolic gives energy by breaking down food into sugar, while a catabolic gives energy by breaking down nutrients that have been stored by the body.* In a sense, one process is healthy and constructive; the other process is unhealthy and can be destructive if the process is continued for a long period of time.

Because the steroid constituents of ginseng are so similar in their structure to the body's own anabolic agents, it is certainly very feasible that they would act in a similar manner.

In addition to its steroid components, ginseng also contains vitamins B_1 and B_2 calcium, postassium, iron, sodium, silicon, magnesium, titanium, barium, strontium, aluminum, manganese, sugar, starch, mucilage, and the following substances that are unique to ginseng:

saponin: the substance that causes the slight foaming when ginseng tea is brewed. A saponin is in the chemical category of glycosides, substances which the body can break down into sugar. It is safe to ingest the saponin in ginseng, but injecting a saponin can have very dangerous effects.

volatile oil: the substance that gives ginseng—especially fresh ginseng—its characteristic odor. The volatile oil of ginseng, sometimes referred to as panasen, evaporates to some extent when the roots are dried out. Some researchers believe that panasen has a direct stimulant effect on the brain, somewhat like caffeine. This substance boils at 105° to 110° Centigrade. It constitutes about 0.05% of the root.

ginsenin: somewhat resembles insulin in its effects. The presence of this substance probably explains the beneficial effect of ginseng in the treatment of alloxan diabetes, in which it is useful. Ginsenin has a glycoside-like chemical structure.

panoxic acid: favorably improves the metabolism and facilitates the efficient functioning of the cardiovascular system. Panoxic acid is actually a chemical mixture of unsaturated fatty acids including palmitic, stearic, oleic, and linoleic acids. Panoxic acid helps prevent the formation of cholesterol, and is thought to facilitate the burning of the body's fat deposits.

panaxin: a substance that has a direct central nervous system stimulant action. It also acts as a tonic to the heart and circulatory system.

panaquilon: a substance believed to stimulate the endocrine system in general, and to maintain proper hormone levels in the body.

strongest

eleutheroside E

eleutheroside C, eleutheroside D

Panaxoside C

eleutheroside B

panaxatriol

eleutheroside F

panaxoside A

panaxadiol

eleutheroside A

panaxoside E

panoxoside F

weakest

Some very interesting and promising results have been obtained by the use of ginseng and *Eleutherococcus* in the treatment of fatigue. One recent study was conducted by the noted pharmacologist, Dr. I. I. Brekhman. A comparison was made of the steroid compounds in the two plants to determine which compounds have the strongest effect in preventing exhaustion following prolonged physical stress.

The chart (opposite) is a comparison of seven steroid constituents of ginseng and six steroid constituents of *Eleutherococcus senticosus*.

On the basis of the preceding chart, it becomes apparent that a need definitely does exist for drug and pharmaceutical firms to seriously look into the possibility of marketing these constituents of ginseng and *Eleutherococcus* individually. At present, it is possible only to obtain ginseng, preparations of ginseng, and preparations of *Eleutherococcus*. There are no companies that sell any of the eleutherosides or panaxosides in pure form; yet these are known to be much more powerful in many respects than the ginseng and *Eleutherococcus* products presently available.

Until the time when these substances are perhaps marketed, we should consider ourselves fortunate indeed that so many high-quality, potent ginseng and *Eleutherococcus* products are readily available.

In some ways, the situation can be compared to that of crude *ma-huang (Ephedra equisetina)* and pure ephedrine (the active ingredient of *ma-huang*). Both have essentially the same medicinal properties; but it is necessary to take a substantial amount of crude *ma-huang*, as compared to very little pure ephedrine, in order to obtain the medicinal effects.

When the constituents of ginseng and *Eleutherococcus* are purified, the dosage will be the equivalent in size of one or two small tablets. This would be equivalent to a much larger amount of the plain roots.

Little-Known Plants That Increase Nonspecific Resistance

By studying 158 folk-medicine preparations used in southeastern Asia, Dr. I. I. Brekhman and his associate, Dr. I. V. Dardymov, were able to uncover some plants that apparently resemble ginseng and *Eleutherococcus* insofar as they are able to increase the nonspecific resistance of the organism to adverse stimuli.

First, they defined these substances to be adaptogens, which must meet the following requirements:

1. They must be virtually non-toxic.
2. They must be nonspecific, increasing resistance in general.
3. They must correct a pathologic condition, yet be unable to worsen any pre-existing pathologic condition.

Within this definition, Brekhman and Dardymov concluded that *Eleutherococcus senticosus* was the strongest adaptogen, followed by *Panax schinseng*. In addition, the following plants were found to have adaptogenic properties:

Rapontium carthamoides	chemical composition unknown
Rhodiola rosea	contains four lactonic substances
Aralia manshurica	contains two aralosides (glycosides of oleanolic acid)
Aralia schmidtii	contains four aralosides
Acanthopanax sessiliflorum	contains four acanthosides, one of which is also present in *Eleutherococcus senticosus*
Kalopanax septemlobum	contains *Kalopanax* saponins

Panaxatriol, from ginseng

Panaxadiol

Cortisone

DCA

Testosterone

Cultivation and Marketing

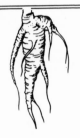

Germination

In nature, ginseng seeds have one of the longest pre-germination dormancy periods known. In other words, after the seeds fall to the ground, there is a very long delay—usually from eighteen months to two years—before the seeds will sprout. Oriental growers of ginseng soon learned, however, that stratification of the seeds would reduce the dormancy period. Under optimum conditions, stratification can reduce the dormancy period to eight months; but it cannot lessen it more than that. In order to stratify ginseng seeds, they are gathered immediately after ripening and stored for several weeks in refrigerated, slightly moist sphagnum moss or other suitable media.

A recent development, even more effective than stratification, is a method that involves the use of a powerful plant hormone, gibberellin. It was found that soaking ginseng seeds in a 0.05 to 0.1 percent solution of gibberellic acid for a day reduces the dormancy period to only six months. Also, the technique seems to greatly increase the number of seeds that will actually germinate. If the method is properly applied, nearly 100 percent of the viable (live) seeds can be induced to germinate in six months. By contrast, using the older methods, only about 60 percent of the viable seeds could be induced to germinate in eight months.

Ginseng Cultivation in Korea

One of the most thorough accounts to date of the details of ginseng cultivation in Korea is provided by George C. Foulk, who wrote the following account in the late 1800s. The general methods in use at that time have changed very little over the years; hence, many of Foulk's observations are still applicable at the present time.

The area of the section at Songto in which ginseng is cultivated is small, not more than eight miles in diameter, and the great majority of the farms are in plain sight from the city, lying about its walls and in the city itself, upon the sights of houses of the time when Songto was the capital of Corea. They appear from the distance as numbers of singular brown patches lying on the grassy slopes rising from the rice paddies. In general, the farms are low, but a few feet above the level of the paddies, but several of the farms I observed were well up on the hillsides.

Each farm is a rectangular compound, one part containing the buildings enclosed by walls, the rest by hedges. The buildings though built as usual of mud, stones, earthenware, and untrimmed timbers, and thatched, are strikeningly superior to the other houses of the Corean people; they are built in right lines, interiors neatly arranged, and walks and hedges in good order. In each compound are one or two tall little watch towers, in which a regular lookout is held over the farm to prevent raids of thieves, who might make off with paying amounts in handfuls of ginseng.

Nearest the entrance to the compound, which is a gate in the buildings court, are guest rooms, where sales are discussed and inspections of the ginseng produced held by officers, and a dry storeroom. Beyond these are two other buildings, in which the curing of the fresh root is carried on; from here on to the end of the compound are parallel rows of low, dark matsheds, with roofs sloping downwards towards the south or southwest. These rows are from 75 to 200 feet high at their front (north) sides, which are closed by mats which swing from the top, thus giving access to the farmer in his care of the plants. Within the sheds are beds about 8 inches high for the growing ginseng plants, which are in two rows extending across the beds, about 2 feet long.

The row (or shed) nearest the houses is the seed bed for all the plants grown on the farm. The soil appeared to be of medium strength as indicated by color, was soft and contained fine granite sand in small proportion (dead leaves broken up finely are used as manure). In the Corean ninth month (September-October) the seeds are stuck quite thickly in the seedbed to a depth of three inches in little watering trenches about three inches apart. Once in each three days' interval during its whole life the plant is watered, and the bed carefully inspected to prevent crowding, decay, and the ravages of worms and insects. The mat-shed is kept closely shut, for ginseng will only grow in the dark or a very weak light.

The mats of the shed are made of round brown reeds and vines closely stitched together, admitting only the faintest light.

In the second month of the second year after planting (February), the root is regarded as formed and the general shape of the plant above ground attained. The root is then tender and white, tapering off evenly from a diameter of three-sixteenths of an inch at the top to a fine long point in a length of 3½ inches; from it hang a number of fine, hair-like tendrils. From the ground stands a single straight reddish stem about two inches, and then spreads out into tiny branches and leaves nearly at right angles to the stem. The shape is nearly that of a matured plant.

In the following February (of the third year), the seed plants are transplanted to adjoining beds, five or six to each cross row, the watering trenches being here between the plant rows. In this second bed the plants remain one year, and are then transplanted to the third bed and planted still farther apart in their respective rows. A year later they are again transplanted, this time to their final beds, where they remain two and a half or three years. Generally speaking, seven years are required from the time of planting until the plant is matured. After its life in the seed bed, exacting care in keeping out the light is not so necessary, and I noticed the swinging mat was removed entirely from the fronts of sheds of plants in the final beds.

In the autumn of the seventh year the seeds ripen and are gathered; these appear on a short stem standing upward from the main stem in continuation of it, where the branches turn off horizontally. The seed stem is broken off an inch above the branches, the seeds sun-dried a little and stored away. Immediately after this the harvest of the roots begins. The seeds are white, rather flat, and round, slightly corrugated, having a diameter of about one-sixteenth of an inch, and a thickness of one-eighth to three-sixteenth inches.

The ripe root has a stem about fourteen inches long, standing nicely perpendicular to the ground. At this distance spread out at a closely common point the branches, usually five, on which, at a distance of about four inches from the main stem top, is a group of five leaves, three large ones radiating at small angles and two small ones at right angles to the branch at their common base. The larger leaves are oval, edges shallowly but sharply notches; length and breadth, 4 and 2 inches respectively; color, nearly a chestnut green. The stem is stiff and woody, ribbed longitudinally. The root is nearly a foot long, and is made up of four different sections ordinarily; the first or upper one, a small irregular knot forming a head to the main root below. From it extends down over the main root a number of slender rootlets terminating in stringy points. The second section is the *body* of the root, which is short, soon separating into a number of bulbous parts, four of which are prominently large. These four parts are commonly called the *legs* and *arms*. The bulbous parts round suddenly and then taper off into small slender sections, from which extends a great number of hairlike feeders. The thickness of the main part of the root or body rarely reaches one inch.

American Ginseng: Cultivated vs. Wild

Although it is universally agreed that wild Oriental ginseng is considerably more valuable than virtually all varieties of cultivated Oriental ginseng, there is no real agreement as to the relative values of wild American ginseng and cultivated American ginseng.

As a rule, wild American ginseng has a much smaller root than the cultivated variety.

In the United States, wild ginseng has been found growing in the approximate region between the Canadian border and the thirty-third parallel; and between the Atlantic Ocean and the Mason-Dixon Line. In other words, it is found primarily in the New England

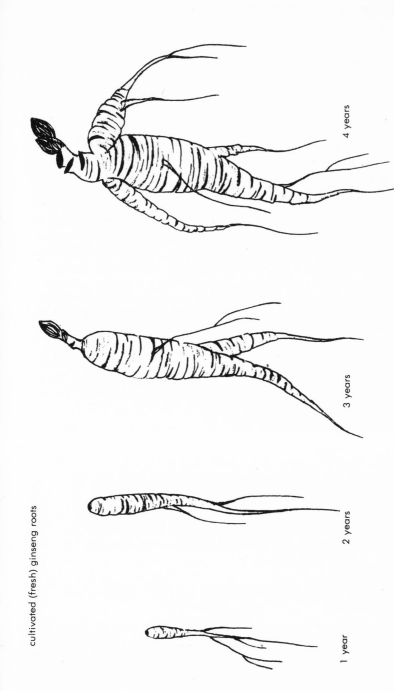

cultivated (fresh) ginseng roots

1 year

2 years

3 years

4 years

111

States, the Great Lakes Region, and the deep South. It can be found growing in many parts of the Canadian wilderness also.

Due to the scarcity of the wild root, however, there is relatively little trade in American wild ginseng. There is certainly not enough to account for any significant part of the ginseng exported to the Orient. For this reason, users of American ginseng in the Orient are familiar only with the cultivated variety and have had no experience with the wild variety. Thus, they would be unable to compare the two forms.

In the United States, there are some ginseng users that believe the wild variety is far more potent than its domestic counterpart. The predominance of wild ginseng in the famous Edgar Cayce formulas seems to imply that this form may be better. Nevertheless, few users of ginseng in the United States are familiar with the wild form, and consequently would be unable to offer an opinion either. It would appear that there is definitely a need for further research into the chemical and pharmacological differences between the wild and cultivated forms.

Wild North American ginseng does cost about twice as much as domestic cultivated ginseng, or Korean ginseng. However, this is a reflection on the scarcity of wild ginseng rather than the demand for it.

Disease of Ginseng

Cultivated ginseng, whether Asian or North American, is highly susceptible to a variety of diseases. Unlike other plants, it is not natural for ginseng plants to grow close together in a crowded situation. In their natural habitat, they are spaced reasonably far apart. In cultivation, the plants are spaced only a couple of inches apart. When a disease organism attacks one plant, it can rapidly spread throughout the entire crop. The natural resistance of the plants is low, so it is relatively easy for an entire crop to be destroyed in a short time.

In Asia, the traditional method of controlling disease consists primarily in repeated transplantation of the plants during their long growing period. When disease breaks out, the diseased plants are immediately destroyed, and the rest of the plants are carefully washed and transplanted. This method is used as often as necessary to prevent the spread of disease. After a crop of ginseng is harvested, the soil is left idle for seven years before replanting. Apparently, whatever organisms are present in the soil that might attack the plants die within the seven year period. This method, though effective, is not highly efficient. It is gradually giving way to more modern methods of disease control.

In North America, many growers lacking ample experience in growing ginseng are at a loss for what to do at the onset of a disease outbreak. A number of fungi can attack the plants. These include *Alternaria panax* (the cause of *Alternaria* leaf spot or *Alternaria* blight), *Phytophthora cactorum* (which attacks the stems and roots), *Rhizoctonia solani* (which attacks the bottom areas of the stems), *Ramularia* spp. (which causes the roots to become rotten), and *Fusarium* spp. (which attacks young seedlings).

Newer methods of disease control are now being tried, and appear to be very promising. Seed disinfection with potassium permanganate or tetramethylthiuram disulfide, and the use of Bordeaux mixture as a spray two or three times during each season have been shown to be an inexpensive and effective means to control the diseases of ginseng.

Profits From North American Ginseng

The market value of North American wild ginseng has consistently remained about twice that of comparable grades of cultivated North American ginseng.

The sale of North American wild ginseng began very soon after the discovery of *Panax quinquefolium* near Montreal in 1716. The roots of the first harvest were sent to China where they were purchased from the collectors at 35 cents a pound. They were subsequently sold in China for a great deal more, and it was not long before the collectors realized that their percentage of profit had been extremely low in this first transaction. The price very quickly rose to about $5 a pound.

About the year 1752, a tragic event took place. Due to an exceedingly large demand for ginseng by the Chinese, North American collectors very hastily gathered the roots in the wrong season, and dried the roots even more hastily. The roots, already too young and immature, were also improperly dried in ovens. So poor was the quality of this shipment that the Chinese refused it altogether. After this, the Chinese tended to mistrust American ginseng. It was not until almost a century later that the market for North American ginseng in China fully recovered.

In the second half of the nineteenth century, the price of North American ginseng steadily rose. During this period, the cultivation of North American ginseng was begun in Virginia in the 1870's. By the beginning of the twentieth century, there were about twenty ginseng growers in the United States, and the market price was roughly $4 a pound.

During the first half of the twentieth century, the market price of North American ginseng seldom ever went below $4 a pound. In fact, it even went as high as $9 a pound.

In 1957, wild American ginseng reached an all-time peak of $24 a pound on the Oriental market.

Since that time, the price on the Oriental market was fluctuated between $15 to as much as $20 a pound.

It should be emphasized that the supply and demand for ginseng are in delicate balance. Although the demand for ginseng remains relatively stable, the supply fluctuates considerably. A very small fluctuation in the supply can, in turn, greatly influence the market price. The current world demand is for approximately 300,000 pounds of ginseng a year. At most, the supply is about 200,000 pounds a year. If the supply were ever to approach the demand, the market price would immediately drop.

Such Forbidding Price

There is no doubt that many non-users of ginseng would try it, and many ginseng users would use it more often, were it not for the characteristically high price of this herb. Actually, the price is only high if viewed relative to most other herbs. If the price of ginseng is compared to many of the proprietary drugs that are on the market, it does not appear any more expensive than many of those.

A prudent buyer will soon learn that some firms ask too much for ginseng products. For example, an herb store in an upper class district will invariably charge more for ginseng than a little shop in Chinatown that caters primarily to Orientals. Of course, this is to be expected. But to find ginseng at a reasonable price, it is not necessary to seek out tiny shops in remote locations. However, it is advisable to shop around and compare prices. Ginseng is not cheap, but you should not pay more than necessary.

One of the main reasons for the high cost of ginseng is the difficulty in growing it, and the length of time involved. The seeds require several months of stratification before they are even planted. If the seeds are treated with gibberellic acid to hasten germination in addition to stratification, they will still require several months after planting before they begin to germinate. After germination, the roots cannot be harvested until they are at least three years old, preferably five or six years old. Also, high initial cost of seeds and susceptibility to disease contribute to a large overhead cost.

Another reason for the high cost is the extreme demand for ginseng in the Orient. To illustrate this point, the lowest grade of cultivated American ginseng roots are purchased in the Orient for a minimum of $9 a pound. Freight and duty charges bring the wholesale price of ginseng sent to the Orient to about $12 a pound.

If Americans do not pay even more than that for ginseng, it is not profitable to sell it domestically. Likewise, it is not profitable for the Orient to export ginseng to the United States if a reasonable profit cannot be made over and above the profit that would be realized by selling it in the Orient.

Because the use of ginseng is much more widespread in the Orient than in the United States, approximately 95 percent of all American ginseng ultimately finds its way to the Orient. Most of it is grown in Marathon County, Wisconsin.

Fraud and Deception

Fortunately, there is probably fairly little real fraud practiced, but the user of ginseng and ginseng products must be aware of some deceptive tactics to watch for. Briefly, they are summarized as follows:

1. Beware of certain types of companies that try to attract potential growers of ginseng. Many of them try to give the impression that

ginseng is easy to grow. On the contrary, it is relatively difficult to grow and subject to many different diseases. Some of them also imply that ginseng can be grown any where in the United States. On the contrary, if ginseng is to be grown outdoors, it can only be grown in the general area in which it has been found in the wild state (or native habitat). In addition to this sort of misrepresentation of the actual facts, these companies often charge enormous prices for seeds and young plants, claiming that your profits will invariably be so enormous that it will pay for the initial investment many times over. This is comparable to selling, for instance, vegetable seeds at an enormous price simply because the vegetable crop will bring in a huge sum of money at harvest time. The logic is absurd. Naturally, the companies that sell ginseng seeds must make a *reasonable* profit, but they have no right to make an exorbitant profit on this premise.

Certainly there are many honest firms that sell ginseng seeds and supplies, but the consumer cannot be too cautious.

2. Another practice, though rare, is to adulterate real ginseng powder with the powdered roots of species such as *Pseudopanax*, *Campanula*, *Adenophora*, and *Platycodon*. All of these plants have roots that resemble real ginseng in color, odor, and appearance. However, they have none of the medicinal properties of ginseng.

If you intend to purchase ginseng powder in any very large quantities, it might be wise to purchase a small amount first and have an analysis done before buying the complete amount. Otherwise, it is probably safer to purchase whole ginseng roots and reduce them to powder using a mortar and pestle or other suitable apparatus.

3. Beware of ginseng roots that are priced extremely low. If you come across ginseng roots priced at, say, $15 a pound, they may have first been used to manufacture ginseng extract, and then dried out. Roots that are extracted in this manner are really worth nothing, because the process of extraction removes all of the active ingredients.

These roots can usually be detected by their bland, dull taste, and their faint aroma. Regular dried ginseng roots should have a fairly strong aroma, and a sharp taste. A regular user of ginseng can immediately recognize the characteristic ginseng odor and taste.

4. Beware of ginseng preparations that do not specify the amount of ginseng they contain. There is no real way to know if such a preparation contains plenty of ginseng, or just a little.

In the past, even more crooked practices than those described above have at least been attempted. George V. Nash, writing in 1898, describes the situation:

> Apart from adulteration there is little fraud practiced except by a few collectors, who load the root with nails, screws, lead, and other heavy substances to make the sample 'weigh up well.' These foreign substances may be inserted while the root is soft with comparative ease. Upon drying, the shrinking of the root generally exposes the metal. Little loss is sustained, however, through this fraud, since the wholesaler refuses such roots as have been plugged, and the country merchant is supposed to shift his prices when bartering groceries and dry goods for ginseng roots.

U.S. Government Publications

At the present time, the U.S. Government offers two small but informative publications that deal with the subject of ginseng:

Ginseng (CA-34-113) is available from: *Letter Sent 2-13-80*

Information Division
U.S. Department of Agriculture
Agricultural Research Service
Federal Center Building
Hyattsville, Maryland 20782

It is a two-page leaflet that gives the basic cultivation requirements of ginseng, currently available at no charge.

Growing Ginseng is available from:

Superintendent of Documents
U.S. Government Printing Office
Washington, D.C. 20402

It is an 8-page, illustrated brochure, revised in 1973. In ordering, be sure to refer to the catalog number (A 1.92201/4) and/or the stock number (S/N 0100-02779), *and* the title. At the present time, this booklet sells for 20¢.

Collection of the Wild Plant

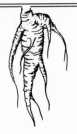

Collection of the Wild Plant

A certain amount of North American ginseng is still obtained by collection of the wild plant. Of course, it is not necessary to gather the roots by yourself. You may, if you wish, purchase roots that have been gathered from the wild, both fresh for planting or dried for medicinal use.

However, if you do wish to gather the root, first be sure that there are no restrictions upon gathering it. In some localities, the plant has wisely been protected by law in order to save it from the threat of extinction.

Refer to the map in this book for the approximate natural habitat of North American ginseng. Within these general boundaries, look for it in shaded woods where the temperature is fairly cool during the summer. In warm areas, it can often be found in the cooler mountain areas at a higher elevation. The plant prefers rich, moist, well-drained soil with an abundance of humus. It is normally found in the shade of such trees as beech, oak, maple, basswood, tamarack, and cedar. It is never found growing in any clearing or in direct sun. Often, a local library will have one or more books on the natural flora of that locality, and this can be extremely helpful in finding the exact location in which wild ginseng can be found.

In gathering ginseng, remember to always leave enough plants to recover growth in that area.

The best time to gather the roots is in late fall, because only at this time can the size of the root be determined by the size of the leaf stalk and the number of berries. Only the plants that are at least three years old should be gathered. If a plant has a stalk that is about eight inches or taller, with two or more leafstalks, it is a fairly good indication that the plant is old enough to be dug. Also, an abundance of berries usually is indicative of an older plant. Very few plants produce any seed at all during the first two years.

The root should be carefully dug and removed in such a way that it is not cut or punctured.

After collection of the roots, remove the stems about half an inch above the root. Then wash the roots very thoroughly, using a non-abrasive brush if necessary. After all dirt has been removed, the roots should be dried either in hot, direct sunlight, or over very low indoor heat. (This heat must not exceed 100°.) In drying the roots, they should always be positioned on racks or cheese cloth mesh to allow for the free circulation of warm air on all surfaces of the root. The racks used, however, must be such that they cannot be corroded by the moist roots. Otherwise, as in the case of iron racks or screens, the roots will pick up a distinct metallic taste. If corrosive metal racks are to be used, they should be covered with cheesecloth or plastic mesh.

In drying ginseng, it is extremely important that the roots become "bone dry." In other words, there must not be any trace of moisture in the root. It is very easy to think that the roots are dry because they appear dry on the outside; whereas they are still quite damp on the inside. If this happens, the root will become moldy in a few days and worthless. This problem is actually peculiar only to ginseng, because ginseng roots cannot be sliced prior to drying without suffering a decrease in value.

After drying, place the roots in a dry, airtight container. Label them with the date gathered and the locality in which they were found.

The native habitat of North American ginseng

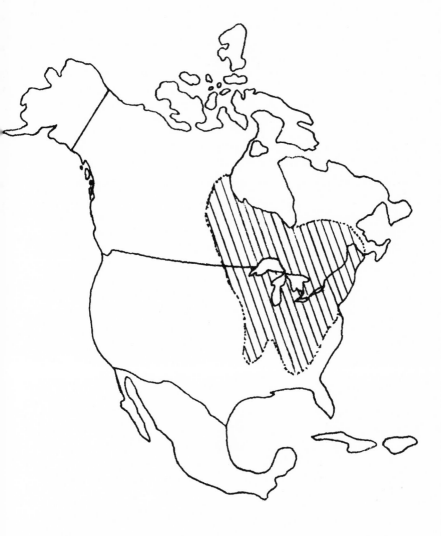

Bibliography

Adams, Samuel Hopkins, 1954. "Treasure Hunt," *The New Yorker*, XXIX, Jan. 16, 1954, pp. 57–63.

Arseniev, V. K., 1939. *Dersu the Trapper*. London: Martin Secker & Warburg Ltd., pp. 10, 85–7, 97, 135, 136, 151–2, 187, 304–5, 341.

Baikov, N., 1936. "Ginseng," *Asia and the Americas*, XXXVI, pp. 601–2.

Ball, James Dyer, 1904. *Things Chinese*. London: John Murray, pp. 316–17.

Bishop, Isabella B., 1897. *Korea and Her Northern Neighbors*. New York: Fleming H. Revell Co., pp. 296–8.

Brekhman, I. I., 1963. "*Eleutherococcus senticosus*—a New Medicinal Herb of the Araliaceae Family," *Proceedings of the 2nd International Pharmacological Congress* (Prague, 1963), vol. VII: "Pharmacology of Oriental Plants." New York: Pergamon Press, pp. 97–102.

Brekhman, I. I., and I. V. Dardymov, 1969. "New Substances of Plant Origin Which Increase Nonspecific Resistance," *Annual Review of Pharmacology*, IX, pp. 419–30.

Brekhman, I. I., 1969. "Pharmacological Investigation of Glycosides From Ginseng and Eleutherococcus," *Lloydia*, XXXII, March, 1969, pp. 46–51.

Bretschneider, E., 1895. *Botanicum Sinicum*, II, p. 105.

————, 1895. *Botanicum Sinicum*, III, pp. 18–25.

Burkill, I. H., 1902. "Ginseng In China," *Kew Bulletin of Miscellaneous Information* (1902), pp. 4–11.

Carney, Frank, 1903. "The Domestication of Ginseng," *The Journal of Geography*, January, 1903, pp. 26–31.

Coe, Charles F., 1904. "Ginseng," *Scientific American Supplement*, LVII, May 7, 1904, pp. 23704–5.

Corlett, William Thomas, 1935. *The Medicine Man of the American Indian and His Cultural Background.* Springfield, Ill.: Charles C. Thomas.

Crane, Louise, 1929. "The Manchurian Man-Image," *Asia and the Americas,* XXIX, pp. 202–7, 234, 235.

Curzon, George P., 1896. *Problems of the Far East.* Westminster: Archibald Constable & Co., p. 168.

Foulk, George C., 1886. "The Ginseng of Korea," *Foreign Relations of the United States* (1886), pp. 328–31.

———, 1887. (Communication No. 275), *Foreign Relations of the United States* (1887), pp. 210–13.

———, 1887. "Note on Korean Ginseng," *Foreign Relations of the United States* (1887), pp. 214–15.

"Ginseng in Smoke," *Business Week,* April 28, 1945, pp. 61–2.

"Ginseng," *Chamber's Journal,* June 8, 1895, pp. 359–60.

Griffis, William Elliot, 1882. *Korea the Hermit Nation.* London: W. H. Allen & Co., pp. 2, 163, 388, 389.

Harding, A. R., 1936. *Ginseng and Other Medicinal Plants.* Columbus, Ohio: Harding Publishing Co.

Harriman, Sarah, 1973. *The Book of Ginseng.* New York: Pyramid Publications.

Harris, Jennie E., 1948. "Stew Me Some Ginseng; I Need Strength," *Natural History,* LVII, Nov. 1948, pp. 424–8.

Heffern, Richard, 1973. *The Herb Buyer's Guide.* New York: Pyramid Publications.

Hibbert, Eloise Talcott, 1941. *Jesuit Adventure In China.* New York: E. P. Dutton & Co., p. 138.

Hoffman, W. J., 1885–6. "The Midewiwin of the Ojibwa," *Annual Report of the Bureau of American Ethnology,* VII, pp. 241–2.

Hosie, Alexander, 1910. *Manchuria.* Boston: J. B. Millet Company, pp. 88–93.

Huc, M. (no date of publication given). *Travels In Tartary, Thibet, and China.* (Translated by W. Hazlitt.) London: Office of the National Illustrated Library, vol. I, pp. 105–6.

Hume, Edward H., 1940. *The Chinese Way In Medicine.* Baltimore: The John Hopkins Press, pp. 145–63.

Jartoux, Father, 1714. "The Description of a Tartarian Plant Called Gin-Seng: With an Account of Its Virtues," *Royal Society of London, Philosophical Translations,* XXVIII, pp. 237–47.

Kains, M. G., 1903. *Ginseng.* New York: Orange Judd Co.

Kirby, E. Stuart, 1971. *The Soviet Far East.* Edinburgh, Scotland: The Macmillan Press.

Lafitau, Father Joseph, 1858. *Memoire . . . concernant la precieux plante du gin-seng.* Montreal: Typographie de Senecal, Daniel et Compagnie.

Lansdell, Henry, 1882. *Through Siberia.* Boston: Houghton, Mifflin & Co., vol. I, pp. 315–6.

Lee, Kyung-Dong, and Richard P. Huemer, 1971. "Antitumoral Activity of *Panax ginseng* Extracts," *Japanese Journal of Pharmacology,* XXI, pp. 299–302.

Lee, Robert H. G., 1970. *The Manchurian Frontier In Ch'ing History*. (Harvard East Asian Series 43) Cambridge, Mass.: Harvard University Press, pp. 87–90.

Millspaugh, Dr. Charles F., 1887. *American Medicinal Plants*. New York: Boericke & Tafel, vol. I, p. 70.

Monachino, Joseph, 1956. "Chinese Herbal Medicine—Recent Studies," *Economic Botany*, X, pp. 42–8.

Mooney, James, 1885–6. "The Swimmer Manuscript," *Annual Report of the Bureau of American Ethnology*, VII, pp. 421–5.

Nash, George V., 1898. *American Ginseng* (U.S.D.A. Division of Botany Bulletin ; 16). Washington, D.C.: U. S. Government Printing Office.

Nickell, J. M., 1972. *J. M. Nickell's Botanical Ready Reference*. Los Angeles: M. L. Baker.

O'Gorman, D. A., 1893. "Ginseng and Its Culture In Korea," *Journal of the Manchester Geographical Society*, IX, pp. 262–3.

Osgood, Cornelius, 1951. *The Koreans and Their Culture*. New York: Ronald Press Co., pp. 19, 91, 129f, 237.

Ossendowski, Ferdinand, 1924. *Man and Mystery In Asia*. New York: E. P. Dutton, pp. 115–20.

Petkov, V., and D. Staneva-Stoicheva, 1963. "The Effect of An Extract of Ginseng On the Adrenal Cortex," *Proceedings of the 2nd International Pharmacological Congress* (Prague, 1963), vol. VII: "Pharmacology of Oriental Plants." New York: Pergamon Press, pp. 39–45.

Pinkerton, John, 1812. *Voyages and Travels*. London: Printed for Longman, Hurst, Rees, etc., vol. 13 "Asia," pp. 639–41.

Pinkerton, Kathrine, 1947. *Bright With Silver*. New York: William Sloane.

Ravenstein, E. G., 1861. *The Russians On the Amur*. London: Trubner & Co., Paternoster Row, pp. 91–2, 253, 309–10.

Semyonov, Yuri, 1944. *The Conquest of Siberia*. (transl. by E. W. Dickes) London: George Routledge & Sons, pp. 305, 308.

Shephard, Dr. I. F., 1884. *United States Consular Reports*. No. 46, XIV, p. 228.

Smith, Huron H., 1933. "Ethnobotany of the Forest Potawatomi," *Bulletin of the Public Museum of the City of Milwaukee*, VII, No. 1, p. 41.

St. George, George, 1969. *Siberia the New Frontier*. New York: Van Rees Press, pp. 119–40.

Swanton, John R., 1924–5. "Religious Beliefs and Medicinal Practices of the Creek Indians," *Annual Report of the Bureau of American Ethnology*, XLII, pp. 485, 511, 656.

Veninga, Louise, 1973. *The Ginseng Book*. Santa Cruz, Calif.: FMALI.

Williams, Llewelyn, 1973. *Growing Ginseng*. (USDA Farmers' Bulletin No. 2201.) Washington, D.C.: U.S. Government Printing Office.

Williams, Louis O., 1957. "Ginseng," *Economic Botany*, XI, p. 344.

Zong, In-Sob, 1952. *Folk Tales From Korea*. London: Routledge & Kegan Paul Ltd., pp. 44–5, 86–8, 166–9.

125

Index

ALPHA BRAIN WAVES
David Boxerman and Aron Spilken
Anyone who has ever heard of meditation, biofeedback or altered consciousness will want to read this fascinating study of the alpha state.
16-0   Paper $4.95

THE COMPLETE BOOK OF ACUPUNCTURE
Dr. Stephen Thomas Chang, Intro. by Dolph B. Ornstein, M.D.
Basic philosophy and practical applications of acupuncture for both laymen and physicians.
124-8   Paper $6.95

THE HEALING ENVIRONMENT
Cristina Ismael
By healing ourselves with and through the environment we begin the process of healing the environment itself.
021-7   Paper $4.95

THE HEALING MIND
Dr. Irving Oyle, Intro. by Stanley Krippner, Ph.D.
Describes what is known about the mysterious ability of the mind to heal the body—through ancient practices that medical science is only beginning to explore, including acupuncture/sonopuncture.
80-4   Paper $4.95

HOW TO GET THE DRAGONS OUT OF YOUR TEMPLE,
Relaxation through Yoga
Diane Neuman
A personal, appealing approach to an ancient technique—a workbook for beginners or those already practicing the pursuit of physical, mental, and spiritual well-being.
118-3   Paper $4.95

THE HUMAN DYNAMO
Hans Holzer
Hans Holzer offers his concepts of a New Age Religion—religious practices that lead to personal fulfillment.
053-5   Paper $4.95

HONG KONG: CUSTOMS AND CULTURE
Duane Rubin
Preface by John H. Pain, Executive Director
Hong Kong Tourist Association
The culture, traditions and customs of Hong Kong made easy for the tourist and arm-chair traveler.
071-3   Paper $4.95

THE REALMS OF HEALING
Stanley Krippner and Alberto Villoldo
Healing and its ramifications, with the "whole person" approach underlying this scientific exploration of one of the world's great "mysteries."
112-4   Paper $6.95